Stransky, Judith.
    The Alexander technique : joy in the
life of your body / by Judith
Stransky, with Robert B. Stone ; ill.
by Shelia Gross; photos. of exercises
by Herb Fogelson. -- New York :
Beaufort Books, c1981.
    x, 308 p. : ill. ; 24 cm.

    Bibliography: p. [301]-302.
    Includes index.
    ISBN 0-8253-0000-2 : $14.95

    1. Alexander technique. I. Stone,
Robert B., joint author. II. Title.

THE ALEXANDER TECHNIQUE

Joy in the Life of Your Body

THE ALEXANDER TECHNIQUE

Joy in the Life of Your Body

by JUDITH STRANSKY

with

ROBERT B. STONE, Ph.D.

Illustrations by Sheila Gross
Photos of Exercises by Herb Fogelson

BEAUFORT BOOKS, INC.
New York   Toronto

Library of Congress Cataloging in Publication Data

Stransky, Judith.
  The Alexander technique.

  Bibliography: p.
  Includes index.
  1. Alexander technique. I. Stone, Robert B., joint author. II. Title.
BF172.S75   1980   158'.9   80-26380
ISBN 0-8253-0000-2

Published in the United States by Beaufort Books, Inc., New York.
Published simultaneously in Canada by Nelson, Foster and Scott Ltd.

Printed in the U.S.A.   First Edition

10 9 8 7 6 5 4 3 2 1

Contents

Foreword by Nina Foch   vii

Introduction   ix

Chapter I   The Alexander Technique—What It Is   1

Chapter II   Free the Body—Free the Person   37

Chapter III   How the Alexander Technique Started   73

Chapter IV   Conditions That Respond to the Technique   87

Chapter V   Meet Your Alexander Teacher— and Be Introduced to Nondoing   110

Chapter VI   Joyous Discoveries You Make   128

Chapter VII   How to Give Yourself Directions: Lying, Sitting, Standing, Walking   162

Chapter VIII   Applying the Language of Good Use   202

Chapter IX   Comparisons, Contrasts, and Similarities of Other Approaches   251

Chapter X   Unveiling the Real You for a Joyous New Life   273

Appendix   299

Bibliography   301

Index   303

Dedicated
to my teachers and colleagues
especially
Judith Leibowitz, Patrick Macdonald, Marjorie Barstow,
Deborah Caplan, Frank Ottiwell,
Virginia Wagner

and to
OTTO

Foreword
by Nina Foch

"Stand up straight!"
"Don't sit like that!"
"Look at your feet!"
"You've got to do something about your posture!"
"Hold yourself up!"
"Pull in your tummy!"
"Don't slouch!"
"Put your shoulders back!"

Half of us have those words in our memories, put there by loving parents, well-meaning relatives, friends who wanted to help. They were no help at all, simply because they pointed out defects but gave no positive method of overcoming them. In our memories, the negatives persist and continue to do harm.

As a teacher of actors, I find that more than fifty percent of my students have posture problems, many of them severe. In youth, these problems may cause only minor discomfort; later, in middle-age and beyond, they lead to real pain.

The usual advice given by acting teachers is to take a dance class: ballet, modern, jazz. All are splendid skills for the actor to have, but none are directed to reeducating the way he or she stands or sits or breathes. What is worse, they are techniques that require conscious thought and we actors have no time to think about posture when we are working. That is too late.

In my own training, I tried every way I could to improve myself, and found that with body and voice the only things that work are techniques that can become a part of your entire life. This is what the Alexander Technique does—better than any technique I know. It has a profound effect on your sense of well-being. Not surprisingly, it makes you feel lighter and more agile, as you are breathing more efficiently. (My husband and son can always tell when I have had an Alexander session; I seem happier, bouyant, less tired.)

By now, you have gathered that I recommend the Alexander Technique not just to actors, but to everyone. It is the *only* effective way I know to reeducate your body, to turn it into your best friend. Judith Stransky has shown me the way. In the five years I have studied with her, I have seen her work miracles with people of all sorts and ages, including young actors, old actors and people with really serious physical problems. Like us, you will be astounded by what simply reeducating the body can do for your sense of well-being and for your effectiveness.

Introduction

"Let the neck be free to let the head go forward and up, to let the back lengthen and widen."

Those words have been said by Alexander teachers all over the world ever since F. Matthias Alexander began to say them to his first students in 1894. Alexander was born in Australia in 1869, and in the 1890's developed a method of body-mind unity, that brings about a joyous self-realization and fulfillment. Alexander was a young actor doing Shakespearean recitations who was confronted with the problem of losing his voice on stage. Physicians could not help him. Instead, he cured himself. First, he observed himself carefully in a mirror and discovered that the way he held his body and used it was causing his vocal problems. He then developed a method of reeducating his body through mental thoughts. The process involved relearning the daily movements of life: sitting, standing, walking, bending, reaching, while using the mental thoughts, "Let the neck be free to let the head go forward and up, to let the back lengthen and widen." He discovered that this psychophysical approach had far-reaching benefits for the whole person—emotional, spiritual, mental and physical. He devoted the rest of his life to teaching others what he had discovered for himself.

Since then, students and teachers of the Alexander Technique—people from all walks of life, ages, and interests—repeat his words in the one-to-one sessions while lying, sitting, moving, and standing. And the back does indeed lengthen and widen as muscles, long accustomed to being tense and tight, are retaught to let go and assume their natural freedom.

With this freedom comes joy—joy beyond belief as the freedom in the body in turn releases the spirit. What a grand feeling to walk tall, physically. It is important. It is therapeutic. But what an even grander feeling to walk tall emotionally and mentally. It is the ultimate in personal restoration and realization.

This book tells you what happens in the Alexander session, a very private session between you and the teacher. It cannot "cause" these benefits to happen to you as you read the book. But it does provide you with valuable new insight into how your thoughts have adversely affected your body and how you may redirect your thoughts to benefit your body. Before you finish this book you will be more aware of your mind-body relationship and you are likely to feel some improvements that bring more life to your body—and yourself.

Who needs the stress that begets more stress? Who needs the muscle tensions that affect vital organs and shorten life? Who needs the everyday body movements that are wasteful, inefficient, and incorrect and only serve to sap energy, depress, and destroy? The answer is, sadly, that some people feel they do. Some people need to bow their shoulders under the weight of the world, for attention, for self-pity.

But the rest of you: follow me. I am an Alexander Technique teacher. My purpose in writing this book is not only to present the story of the Alexander Technique to you but to give you an actual feeling of it so that you can begin to move in a more natural way toward better health, greater physical attractiveness, and a higher level of emotional well-being.

The prize at the end of the road is the joy of expressing yourself in a way that you may have dreamed about but found to be an impossible dream, leaving you frustrated and hopeless.

I once felt that frustration. Now I feel the joy.

I want to share it with you.

I will show you the way toward liberation from old, unwanted conditionings. It is an easy way, a remarkable way. It is certainly a unique way—to a joy and a life beyond belief.

THE ALEXANDER TECHNIQUE: an effortless mind-body experience that unlocks the flow of physical, mental, and spiritual energy to higher levels of well-being and effectiveness. Thanks to this decades-old teaching procedure, recently come of age, thousands are enjoying renewed youth, health, vitality, attractiveness, and peace of mind.

Chapter 1

The Alexander Technique— What It Is

A YOUNG MAN is seated. A woman is standing beside the chair, facing him. She has one hand placed lightly under his chin. The fingers of the other hand are gently touching the back of his head.

"Forget about standing up, Paul. Leave it up to me to get you up out of the chair. Instead of thinking about getting up, I would like you to say these words to yourself: *Let the neck be free, to let the head go forward and up, to let the back lengthen and widen.*

"As you say these words over and over to yourself, imagine that your head is floating up to the ceiling." If you were the teacher, your hands would detect a light, upward energizing sensation in Paul's body before he has even finished thinking that thought.

When the teacher feels that signal, she moves Paul easily up from the chair to a standing position as if he were feather-light. This is not, however, his usual standing posture. His shoulders are not hunched and his whole body, from head to heels, is in good alignment, yet without any apparent effort on his part.

Paul had been plagued with spells of pain in his upper back between the shoulder blades. Now that he has had several lessons in the Technique, he is unlearning the poor standing and sitting habits he had developed over the years and learning how to release the tensions that they had caused.

Paul is one of the thousands of people who take lessons in the Alexander Technique. Many come to acquire better posture, grace of movement, and physical attractiveness. But many come because of physical disorders such as backaches, migraine headaches, arthritis, asthma, gastrointestinal problems, high blood pressure, and respiratory ailments. Others come because of emotional problems, such as chronic depression, feelings of inferiority or sexual failures.

The people who come include people in the performing arts, the professions, and all walks of life. Said Princess Lee Radziwill about the Alexander Technique in an interview, "You do no real exercise, yet you come out feeling as if you're breathing and moving correctly for the first time. Like a dancer."*

Medical practitioners regularly refer patients to Alexander Technique teachers, usually with the same positive results recently expressed by Professor Nikolaas Tinbergen, co-winner of the 1973 Nobel Prize for Medicine. Speaking about himself and his family, he said, "From personal experience we can already confirm some of the seemingly fantastic claims made by Alexander and his followers, namely, that many types of underperformance and even ailments, both mental and physical, can be alleviated, sometimes to a surprising extent, by teaching the body musculature to function differently. . . . We already notice, with growing amazement, very striking improvements in such diverse things as high blood pressure, breathing, depth of sleep, overall cheerfulness and mental alertness, resilience against outside pressures, and also in such a refined skill as playing a stringed instrument."**

A 52-year-old psychotherapist, crippled from polio in his legs and suffering severe pains in his back came to me for lessons. It was quite a challenge—not only to me, but also to the Alexander Technique. He had misgivings about the visit: "When I came to your office and lay down upon your table, the phrase 'an exercise in futility' ran through my mind," he wrote to me after his first lesson. Here is how he described the change that took place within a half hour:

"When I left I was in 75% less physical pain. I was no longer angry. I felt lighter and more in control of my body. I walked to my car, opened the door and got in effortlessly. My posture was better all the way home. It was indeed a pleasure!"

*McCalls, February, 1968

**"Ethology and Stress Diseases," speech reprinted in Science, July 5, 1974.

Here is how a 45-year-old housewife describes what happened to her:

"As I told you, I was in constant pain between the shoulders and the upper back. One lesson, and the pain left. Since major abdominal surgery thirteen years ago, I have had to wear firm, boned girdles from morning to bedtime because of intense lower back pain. I did not wear my girdle after the Alexander lesson. In the past it would have been impossible for me to scrub or iron without the girdle. That night, after driving one hundred miles—usual duties for a six-member family—I was able to scrub, vacuum, wash, and iron clothes for one-and-a-half hours. I felt like I was really floating!"

A well-known award-winning New York dress designer suffered from severe back pains. She was constantly on the run working for three different companies. She also went weekly to the famous Kounovsky's gym in Manhattan. She was a former ballet dancer, and had the tight sway back, tilted pelvis, tense buttocks, and turned out legs so common among them.

She came for Alexander lessons twice a week. An immediate result was less back pain; after a few weeks there was no pain whatsoever. She continued the lessons, realizing that more lessons were required for a lasting change in her body posture and functioning. One day she reported that she and her husband had taken their annual walk across the Brooklyn Bridge, a fairly long hike. "I always used to be sore the next day. Not so this time. No soreness at all. In fact, the next day I felt that I could do it all over again."

After a few months, her gym instructor told her that her back was far improved. "Your back used to be so bad that I was afraid you would damage it while doing some of the gymnastics," she was told.

After some months of Alexander lessons, she took a ballet class again, and reported to me that her muscles did not ache the next day, even though she had not had a class for more than a year. In the past, if she had missed only one week of class, her muscles would be very sore the day after her next class.

Now she had an awareness of her body and of her capacities. She could sense when she had done enough of a particular movement and now avoided overdoing it. Compared to the past, when everything had been difficult and a strain, all she did now seemed easy.

One year after she had commenced the lessons she confided to me that she was pregnant. "You are the first to know, even before my husband. Without your lessons I would never have had children—I had seen my mother with terrible back pain during her pregnancies, and I had seen her wear ugly supportive lace-up corsets. I had decided I would never go through that."

She continued her lessons once a week throughout her pregnancy, without a hint of back pain, and looked barely pregnant.

During this period she had been appointed special designer for one of the most glamorous department stores in New York. In her eighth month of pregnancy, she had her first showing. She sailed easily through the work and the pressures.

After her child was born, she had a few more lessons. She lost her extra weight very rapidly, and her figure was better than ever. She then discontinued the lessons, feeling no need for more. When I saw her two years later, her figure was superb, she was radiant and pain-free, and thrilled with the results of the Technique and its long-lasting effect. Soon after she became pregnant again and went easily through her second pregnancy, childbirth, and post-child-birth.

The Alexander Technique is *not a cure*. It is *not a treatment*.

The Alexander Technique is a series of lessons that *teaches you how to move* in all activities, from the simplest to the most complex, in the most natural and easy manner. It teaches you a basic pattern of good use, which gradually becomes your natural and constant way of moving. It teaches you to unlearn the poor habits that you have developed, caused by tension and causing more tension, and to experience again the free, easy and natural way of moving that you once had before the poor habits set in.

Just What Does A Person Learn Through the Alexander Technique?

An Interview with Judith Stransky, Alexander Teacher.
Reprinted from *Bulletin of Structural Integration*, Winter, 1969-70.

What you learn in the Alexander Technique is a grace, flexibility, and ease that you apply constantly to everything that you do. This is as opposed, say, to the grace and flexibility learned in dancing which are not (necessarily) applied to daily life. One of the most remarkable results is the sensation of lightness that students experience after lessons, and that stays with them almost constantly. Another is lessening of fatigue.

These feelings are the result of learning to use oneself well, which involves improved alignment and posture. Essentially, habits are changed. Correct alignment and improved use are achieved by eliminating incorrect use and good habits are substituted for bad ones. When learning good use you must first stop the cycle of deterioration, and you then start a new cycle of good use.

Q: *How do the lessons begin? Is there a diagnosis of the student's specific needs?*

A: For each student the lesson is conducted in essentially the same way, because essentially we are teaching good use, we are not treating specific problems. In diagnosing a person's problems—his misuse or poor alignment—the teacher not only observes with the eye, but also feels the tension with his hands.

Q: *Why do people come for lessons, generally?*

A: People come because of pain or discomfort; they also come to improve posture. Others come for professional reasons, such as dancers, actors, musicians . . . they learn to use themselves well in their daily lives, and this basic good, free use of their bodies enables them to perform better and to be less fatigued. But anyone could benefit from lessons. For example, say an alto saxophone player came for lessons. In a short time he has better alignment, he uses his body better, his breathing improves, and more energy is available to him. I once saw this demonstrated in a dramatic way at a lecture on the Alexander Technique in New York. The teacher took someone from the audience who had never had an Alexander lesson and demonstrated: with the hands on the head and neck she gave the orders and took the person in and out of the chair very easily, and the whole alignment changed. It was obvious to the whole audience. It couldn't have happened without the touch of the teacher's hands, true, but the participant had to give the order to release as well, and then the release *happened*. You need both the order from the student and the teacher's hands guiding the student into a good direction. In repeated lessons we are actually influencing or re-conditioning reflexes through repeated sensory experience together with verbal commands.

Q: *Just for clarification, how do you use the term, "conditioned reflex"?*

A: If a person sits down in a chair he is going to use certain habits to accomplish that act. His muscles will function in a certain way. That's his conditioned reflex at that time. Now in the Alexander lessons, we change that for the better, so that his reflex response to the thought, or the order, of sitting will be a different response. He will use his muscles in a different way, possibly even use different muscles.

Q: *How do you get around the problem which is often foreseen, of simply substituting another pattern, that the student may have to unlearn later?*

A: There are two issues involved here. One is the question of the reeducation (or reconditioning) itself, and how it is done. I will go into a whole explanation of the lesson and what happens in a lesson. But before I do that I think I should answer your question about imposing another conditioning on top of one that is already there. The way I see it is that you are unlearning, rather than learning something new. You are unlearning poor habits, poor responses, so that you can come to relearning the original good use: good responses to orders, wishes, and desires. That's why Alexander calls it a *re*-education rather than an education, because reeducation implies that you are learning something that you once knew.

Now then, the second question, how is this done?

In the lessons, first of all, the student is asked to do nothing. Even if I want the student to sit down on a chair, I don't want him to *do* it. He has to leave himself alone entirely, and let me move him. We are not super-imposing something on top of the habits that he already has; we are stopping him from using the habits he has. He is to be free, open, and neutral in order to experience something else. What he is going to experience is the way he used to function once upon a time, before the poor habits took over.

Q: *What are the most common barriers that you encounter with students?*

A: In the beginning the greatest difficulty is for people to do nothing—to simply lie still on the table, or sit still in the chair, or stand still. When I give them the verbal orders, "Let the neck be free to let the head go forward and up, to let the back lengthen and widen," their greatest difficulty is simply to be still, and to say the words to themselves *without doing anything muscularly.* Even if they don't know what those words mean, it is as if they start moving muscles by reflex. They immediately want to start to "do" something about it. They are usually not aware that they are "doing" something. But with my trained and experienced eye I can see it, and with my hands I can feel it. For example, I may have my hand on the knee when a person is sitting in the chair and I will feel that the person has the impulse to move his head and neck, or move an arm. One can feel it throughout the whole organism if one is sensitive to it, and trained to feel it. In the beginning the student is usually not aware that he has made a slight movement; it is reflex response for him; he is not aware that he has done it.

Then we reach a stage in the work where the student becomes aware that he has moved; he may not be able to prevent it yet, but he becomes aware *when* he has moved. Then follows the stage where he can prevent it. He can stop himself from actually making a movement. He can just give the directions and be still, which is what Alexander called "inhibition"; that is, inhibition in the best sense of the word, when one inhibits harmful "doings" and makes the choice to substitute improved use. When the student reaches that stage, we get to the more individual problems of the person. One person will have greater tension, greater holding in the head-neck area, another will have it in the chest area, another in the abdominal area, another in the legs or the pelvic area, and the hip joints. Now I may observe in the beginning where the greatest tension is. But until the student learns to "leave himself alone" he is not aware of it himself as a rule. What often happens is that as the student becomes freer he is able to release in the area where the strongest holding is. No sooner has he done this than we become aware of other areas that are tense and they eventually release as the lessons progress.

There is always head-neck tension if there is tension in any part of the body. This is a uniform pattern. If one tenses anywhere in the organism, the head-neck area will become tense simultaneously. Aside from this universal head-neck tension, which is present in almost everyone to some degree, I find that one of the greatest areas of holding and of tension is in the area of the rib cage. This is directly related to breathing, of course. I think everyone is aware nowadays, that good breathing is essential to the proper functioning of the various systems of our bodies. We don't work with breathing itself. We don't prescribe breathing exercises, or anything like that, but we find that as the alignment improves, as the musculature around the rib cage releases, and allows a freer rib cage, then the breathing improves naturally. We work for organic rather than mechanistic changes in the body's functioning.

Q: *How would you describe or define "organic change?"*

A: By organic I mean—evolutionary—that it happens gradually and synergistically. You see, so many things are dependent on each other, that we work with the total organism instead of working on particular parts or particular problems. We work with the pattern of the whole organism, which is based upon the alignment of the head, neck and torso. Now if a person has tight legs, I'm not going to spend a lot of time trying to get those legs free. It is possible for me to help the person to have the experience of his legs moving freely, but if his head, neck and torso are not free, the moment I take my hands away from his legs or the moment he makes a move on his own, he'll tighten up immediately. On the other hand, if there is a release in the head, neck and torso area, his legs will release automatically to a certain degree. I am not saying they will release one hundred percent, because muscles can have stiffened over the years from not having functioned freely, so that it will take a little time. They need the experience over and over again of functioning freely, and then will gradually they come back to their full, free use.

Q: *The relationship of head, neck, and torso was what Alexander was referring to in the term "primary control?"*

A: That's right. What he actually was referring to when he said "primary control" was the relationship of the head to the spine—whether that relationship is good or bad, that *is* the "primary control"! If that relationship is poor, the functioning of the rest of the organism will be poor. In the term "primary control" Alexander was referring not only to the relationship of the head to the spine, but that the head has to be poised lightly on top of the spine *to allow* it to lengthen. That indicates to me that you are actually controlling the way you function, whether you are at rest or in movement. Also, the term "primary control" gives a picture of the head literally leading everything. This seems logical and in order. Again, let it be understood, that when Alexandrians use the term "control" it is not meant as a muscular control which would involve rigidity or forcing. The control comes through thinking. I want to stress this. Alexander often used a phrase to describe his technique: "psycho-physical reeducation with conscious control in the use of the self." The term "conscious control" is a key term; it means that you control through thinking—through conscious thoughts. You control with your brain, which is in your head. It's not in your pelvis, and it is not in your solar plexus. There are many methods of dance and body movement, etc., which have similar ideas of what good alignment is, but they think of it as starting from the pelvis—that the pelvis has to be in a certain relationship with the rest of the torso, and they ignore the head. I think this is limiting. I think that they do get some results. In some cases they get very good results, but I don't think they always get their maximum result because they are leaving out the concept that Alexander found—that your brain is going to control everything by the way it gives orders to the organism, and that the head leads the torso upwards.

Q: *Changing the subject a bit, what is the teacher's part in this kinesthetic reeducation? I mean, is it not possible for the student to work on his own?*

A: To put it most simply, the feelings we have when we are misusing ourselves are not reliable. Let me give you an example. A man comes in for lessons and one shoulder is much lower than the other. He has been walking around like this half of his life, and he doesn't feel that it is lower. It feels "normal" to him. Now let's say that I got his shoulders to level out. He would look level but he would not feel level. That is why he needs a teacher to help him to achieve a state of good balance, and symmetry, and he needs a mirror to see that it *is* that way, because his feelings are going to tell him that it isn't that way.

Q: *But obviously Alexander didn't have a teacher . . .*

A: Alexander was a genius in the respect that he could do it for himself, but it took him nine years of painstaking observation and study, working with himself in front of a three-way mirror. Through observing himself, he started observing other people, and he saw that most people had the same kind of problem. In the last analysis there are probably some people who could "teach themselves" but most people would not be that persistent.

Q: *Doesn't it seem remarkable that he, never having experienced these sensations at the hands of anyone else, could devise a technique for communicating so much information?*

A: Yes. Alexander was an unusual man. I have been told by people who studied with Alexander personally that the touch was incredibly light, yet remarkable things happened. They described his touch as "soft as lambswool" or "soft as butter." Alexander apparently really was able to pass across the very essence of his work.

Q: *And what do you think that essence was?*

A: I think it was Nondoing. Through a light touch, with no force, no strong manipulation, you can bring about changes.

Q: *This point will be interesting to many of our readers. Would you describe these changes also as* structural *changes?*

A: Yes, they are structural changes, and this is very obvious when we observe the student in the mirror. I work in front of a mirror with the student so that he can see the changes happening during a lesson. Also I take photographs of the student when he first comes for lessons, and then some weeks or months later when I think there is an obvious change. When we compare them we can see the gradual change in the person's posture and alignment. There is definitely a structural change, it is obvious during the lessons, and it is obvious over a period of time. Students find friends and relatives noticing and saying "Oh, you look much taller," or "You look thinner," yet they may not have lost an ounce; it is simply that they are carrying themselves in a more superb manner. Yes, there is definitely a structural change, but it is not done through forcing. It is really that my hands are guiding. Another way of putting it is that my hands stimulate a person to go into the direction of lengthening. The stimulus comes both from the thoughts that we think (the verbal directions that we give), and the teacher's hands touching the student to add to the stimulus, and, when necessary to inhibit the incorrect response.

Simple Ways to Get the Alexander Technique Feeling

Let's do a little experiment.

Sit on a chair the usual way and stand up as you always do. Stand up and sit down a few times, without trying to change the way you usually do it.

SITTING TO STANDING

GOOD USE

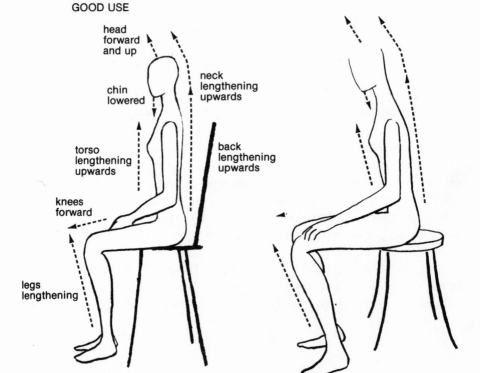

head forward and up

neck lengthening upwards

chin lowered

torso lengthening upwards

back lengthening upwards

knees forward

legs lengthening

Can you feel which parts of your body are working the hardest? Is it your neck, or your shoulders, or your lower back; your thighs, or calf muscles, or feet? Is it several of these, or all?

See if you can sense whether you throw your head backwards—even if it is only slightly—and push your chin upwards in the air, as you sit down and stand up. Do you feel the back of your neck tightening?

Now I would like to show you another way.

Sit down again. Drop the chin a little bit, as if you are nodding "yes" to someone. Leave the chin at the bottom of the nod. Begin telling yourself easily that your head is floating upwards toward the ceiling. Say it to yourself over and over again, while you are looking downwards.

Don't try to have your back straight up. Instead, let your head and torso lean forward slightly.

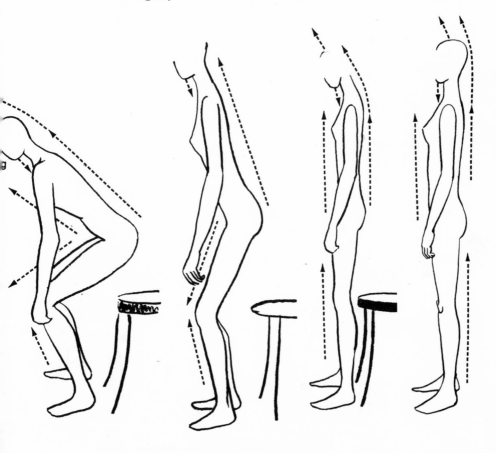

Now, continuing to lower your chin, and still saying over and over again that your head is floating upwards, lean a little further forward and allow yourself to rise up to an easy standing position.

Do you feel easier? Was there less tension in the neck, back and shoulders? Perhaps you felt your legs working harder. If so, that is good. It means that your back was not taking over a job that does not belong to it. Your back muscles were lengthening and supporting the spine, shoulder blades, neck and skull, as they are supposed to do. Therefore, the legs were doing the work *they* were supposed to do. Today, they aren't used to it. Soon it will be effortless.

Now you are standing up. Before sitting down again drop your chin slightly into the bottom part of the "yes" nod, look downwards, and *think* of moving your head upwards as before. Again, please do *not* try to keep your back straight. Now, while *thinking* of your head constantly moving upwards, let your knees and hip joints bend

SITTING TO STANDING

POOR USE

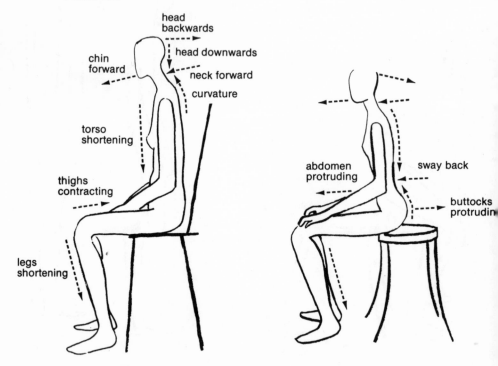

head backwards

chin forward

head downwards

neck forward

curvature

torso shortening

thighs contracting

legs shortening

abdomen protruding

sway back

buttocks protruding

gradually—still lowering your chin and telling your head to go upwards—until you feel the chair under your buttocks.

Your back did not feel straight, did it? Your head and torso leaned forward a little. That's fine. Let them do what feels natural and easy (not stiff) as you go to the chair. You have to bend your knees and hip joints to reach the chair. All the way down, keep on lowering your chin without permitting the neck to drop forward as it might tend to, and tell your head to float up towards the ceiling. "See" your head floating up, at a slight forward angle.

Try this a few times. The most essential thing is not to attempt to keep your back straight. Just let the movement happen easily. And repeatedly tell your head to move upwards.

➡ How to Size Yourself Up

Stand sideways in front of a mirror. Turn your head slowly to the

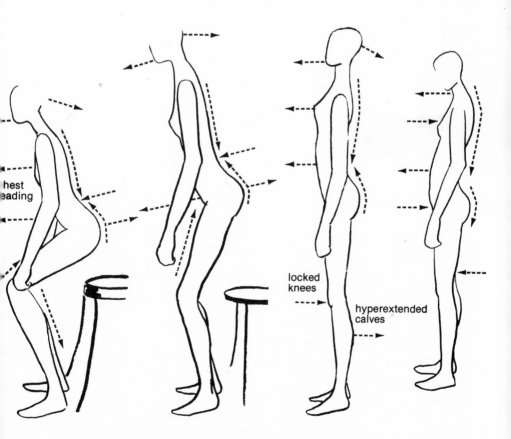

side and look at your profile. Do you have rounded shoulders and a hunched-over curve in the upper back? Do you have a sway back, curving at the midsection? Do you have both?

Turn your head away from the mirror to the front. Now straighten up. Glance sideways into the mirror. Are you really straight, or are. you standing with more of a sway back? Are your shoulders pulled backwards? Is your head pulled backwards? Do you feel comfortable or do you feel strained and unnatural?

Now perhaps you look more upright in the mirror. But are you comfortable? Do you feel natural?

Look very carefully at your head. Is it really going upwards? Or is it going backwards and downwards?

HEAD-NECK RELATIONSHIP

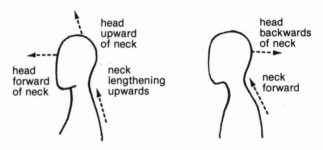

head
upward
of neck

head
forward
of neck

neck
lengthening
upwards

head
backwards
of neck

neck
forward

Look at the rest of your body in the mirror. Observe your neck, back, shoulders, buttocks, legs. How do they look to you?

Now let's do something with the head. Face front again, so that you are not looking in the mirror, and purposely push your head backwards and downwards, so that your chin is sticking up towards the ceiling. What can you sense in the rest of your body as a result of what you've just done? Do you sense that the back of your neck is shortened and tighter? Do you sense that your spine is more compressed and more stiff? Do you feel that there is some tension in your buttocks? What about tension in your hip joints? How about your legs? Perhaps you feel that there is a lot of pressure on the feet, that they are pressed down into the floor.

Now turn your head to the mirror and look at your profile, and see if you can notice any of that effect. Do your shoulder blades stick out more in the back? Do you have more of a sway back? Does your pelvis stick out more behind? Are your legs straight, or are they at an angle?

Don't stay long in that position, because it is a strain. People who do this constantly can develop severe back pains. Turn your head to the front again, and let your head come back to what feels normal to you.

Now let's do something that is different to what you have just done. Push the top of your head upwards toward the ceiling. Make yourself as tall as possible. Stretch your back upwards.

You can pretend that a string is pulling your head up towards the ceiling and stretching your spine and back. What does that feel like? It probably is quite a strain, particularly in the back of the neck. Does the back of your neck feel strained and pulled upwards in an uncomfortable manner? Perhaps your whole spine feels uncomfortably pulled upwards.

Now slowly turn your head, keeping the upward stretch, to look in the mirror and see what effect that head position has on the way you are standing. Your back may look straight in the mirror. It is quite possible that now you have no abnormal curves in the back and neck, and that your back and your legs are straight. Take note of your breathing and how your chest and throat feel. Do you notice that your breathing is more difficult, and your chest quite rigid, your throat tight, and your legs strained?

Now turn your head again to the front and let go of the pushing upwards. You probably feel quite relieved at not having to push your head backwards and downwards, or upwards. Probably your breathing is easier.

By pushing your head upwards and forcing yourself to stretch upwards and be as tall as possible, you can improve the look of your posture. You can make yourself *look* much straighter, but it is done at the expense of straining muscles, which is a very unnatural condition. Should you continue to do that for any length of time, you could end up with a pain in the back of the neck.

Some people do this habitually. They are, usually, very stiff and rigid people. They cannot move or breathe freely. Usually they are not spontaneous and free in their behavior either. In fact, they are the kind of people you might say are a pain in the neck.

▶ The Body and The Mind: A Symbiotic Partnership

Body types and personalities are interrelated. Personality can be strikingly influenced by the body's posture. The person who is slumped down tends to be depressed and lethargic.

It also works the other way around. Certainly you have experienced times when you felt very happy and joyous, and your body also felt light and buoyant, and straighter. Later that feeling disappeared and you wondered why you couldn't always feel that good. Mood affects body, and body affects mood. When you haven't exercised in a long time, you feel sluggish and low, and not only in the body. Then one day you swim, hike, jog, run, or do some type of exercise, and you feel exhilarated in spirit as well as body.

What the Alexander Technique does is teach you to achieve that wonderful feeling and have it all the time. And though the degree will vary, you will never go all the way down into the dumps again, or feel as stiff, awkward and heavy as you did before.

Now let's try something that may give you a taste of that light feeling. Stand again so that you can see your profile in the mirror. Look straight ahead. Now lower your chin a little bit. (But *don't* drop your neck forward.) Do it as if you are slightly nodding "yes" to someone, easily. Leave your chin in the downward part of the "yes" nod.

While you do that, *think* of your head as a balloon. *Think* of it floating up towards the ceiling, and pretend that there is a slight breeze behind it wafting the balloon slightly forward as it floats upward, so that it reaches the ceiling, touching it lightly about two or three inches forward of the spot right above your head. This is the direction we call "Head forward and up."

While you think of your head going "forward and up," think of your back and spine as being very long, following the head upwards. DO NOT DO ANYTHING. DO NOT SAY ANYTHING OUT

_OUD. Just *think* these directions. Say them silently to yourself. It s very important—in fact, it is essential—that you do *not* try to *do* ıny movements in these directions, except for that slight downward ıod, which releases the neck muscles in the back, *allowing* the head o go forward and up and the back to lengthen upward.

Stand in a normal position while you visualize the lengthening ıpwards. Don't slump, and don't try to stand up straight.

Instead, stand in a natural position, with your chin in that slight ıod and think about your head floating "forward and up," like a ›alloon. Think of your spine, back and neck as being made of elastic ¡hat is stretching upwards. They are attached to the balloon. The top ·f your neck is attached to the balloon, and as the balloon floats ıpward toward the ceiling your neck, back and spine are all gently ¡tretched upwards (in your thoughts), and "lengthened." Although ·ou are only thinking this, you might feel a slight upwards move-¡nent and a sensation of being lighter. Think these thoughts fre-¡uently and rapidly, as if it is a game. *Don't get serious.* That will ¡nake you hold your breath and feel stiff. Play with these thoughts ¡ghtly over and over again.

Now, together with these thoughts we can say the words that ılexander himself used and that Alexander teachers apply to this ay:

"LET THE NECK BE FREE, TO LET THE HEAD GO FORWARD AND UP, TO LET THE BACK LENGTHEN AND WIDEN."

Say these words to yourself effortlessly and rapidly, over and over. ¦ven try putting a little rhythm into it, as if it is a little song or a ·oem. *Lightly. Playfully.*

Again, say the words casually over and over again:

> *"Let the neck be free,*
> *Let the head go forward and up,*
> *Let the back lengthen and widen,*
> *Let the neck be free,*

Let the head go forward and up,
Let the back lengthen and widen . . ."

▶ Thinking the Words

There is absolutely nothing else to do. Merely say these words.
imagine the thoughts, and don't make any changes. Be neutral.

While saying these words, you may sense some very slight, subtle
changes or sensations in your body. These sensations may feel new to
you, or they may remind you of some similar sensations you have
sometimes had in the past. You might say to yourself: "I'm not sure if
I'm feeling anything or not. There is something going on, but I think
it's my imagination."

So many students have said that to Alexander teachers after they
started to experience the Alexander Technique, that we know it is
not their imagination. Whatever you feel so slightly is actually
happening. Gently turn your head and look in the mirror—perhaps
there is some change in the way you are standing.

Think these thoughts and say these words from now on any time
you want to, and see what it feels like. Do it *only by thinking the
thoughts* and saying the words to yourself in your mind *without*
trying to bring about any change, or moving muscles in any special
way.

It is important to give yourself the directions with eyes open.
Students are asked to do this during Alexander lessons. Look ahead
in a natural way. Or, drop your eyes a little, as if you are looking at
something on the ground in the far distance. Blink your eyes normally to avoid staring. Notice your breathing. See that you are not
holding your breath. Don't do anything special about your breathing; simply notice that it's happening. Try the directions again, being
aware of your eyes and your breathing. Don't work at any of this, and
please don't make an effort.

The Alexander directions are effective only when you apply them
in the most natural state—without staring, holding the breath, or
going into a special state of "concentration."

What you learn in the Alexander Technique is to move freely and
well and easily in your daily life. It is not something to be practiced at

a set time. We apply the Alexander Technique to our daily lives, standing... sitting... walking...

▶ Feeling the Benefits of the Alexander Technique in a Chair

Now try these Alexander instructions—the words and the thoughts—sitting on a chair.

Sit about half-way forward on the chair, your knees and feet fairly wide apart, your feet on the floor. Again, drop your head ever so slightly into that little "yes" nod. Again, *think* of your head floating up towards the ceiling like a balloon, forwards and upwards, and *think* of your back and neck also going up becoming as long as possible, like malleable elastic.

While giving the directions, let your eyes blink normally while looking ahead (not down), and let your breathing be normal. See if you sense any kind of sensation in your body as you think these "directions" while sitting. Do you find it easier to give these directions and do nothing while you are sitting compared to when you are standing? Many people find it difficult or even impossible to stand without making some effort to keep themselves standing. (Until, that is, they have had some Alexander lessons.) They find it easier to sit. With others, it is the reverse.

Say the words, "Neck free, head forward and up, back lengthening. Neck free, head forward and up, back lengthening. Neck free..." Say them as many times as you like, without a care in the world.

Do you sense some slight sensation of lightening, perhaps of lifting off the chair? Perhaps you sense that your shoulders are softening and easing up? Perhaps your head feels very light. Note any sensations you may have similar to any of these. (Electromyograph machines have recorded muscular movement when a subject merely *thinks* of moving a particular part of the body.)

In an actual Alexander lesson, you the student have the benefit of the teacher's hands touching you lightly in the head-neck-back areas, moving you up from the chair to a standing position, or down to the chair to sit. The instructor will move you to bend, reach for things, pick things up from the floor, or reach for something above you. You will stand on your toes, bend your knees, learning different kinds of bends for different kinds of activities—you will be walking, standing, lying down, moving your arms, moving your legs, all with the lightest touch from the teacher's hands. You will be working with the movements of your daily life.

On your own, you will get benefits from using these Alexander "directions" (the thoughts and words). These benefits will be in proportion to the frequency and to the multiplicity of activities and occasions that you think of them.

Here are some of the sensations that turn into real benefits:
- Lightness
- Ease
- More vitality
- Lighter head
- Freer neck
- Lighter, longer back
- Release in the shoulders
- Release in the buttocks
- Release in the legs
- More joy

Maybe you have just felt all of these things, or maybe it was a sensation that you can't describe. Some say they feel as if they have just meditated. Some people say they feel stoned, as if they had taken drugs. Some say it is the same sensation as they get from T'ai chi. Or they may compare it with what they have felt from some other technique that releases a natural ease in the body.

When you have the assistance of the Alexander teacher, you feel light, buoyant and easy more constantly than when you "practice" on your own. Still, the benefits you receive on your own are worth many times over the brief moments required to think the directions.

With the delicious sensations, there comes a glowing change in appearance. Alexander students look brighter, more vital, more youthful. They move with ease and grace. Their bodies are better aligned.

They become better proportioned—waists become more slender,

chests and shoulders broader, bosoms uplifted. Their legs are straighter, feet stronger, muscles strengthened.

Their posture improves without effort. They have an air of assurance, of a joyous floating through life.

➡ The Alexander Teacher and You

Let's go back to Paul. I am Paul's teacher.

When I give him the instructions to think, "Let the neck be free, to let the head go forward and up, to let the back lengthen and widen," I immediately feel something. Remember, I have one hand placed lightly under his chin, the other at the back of his head with some fingers lightly touching the back of his neck.

As Paul thinks these thoughts, before he has even finished thinking them, I feel a light, upward, energizing sensation in his body. It is almost as if my hands are an electromyograph.

At that moment, I start to move him easily out of the chair until he is standing. The process of moving up out of the chair to a standing position used less energy than it normally did. The result is that he stands before the chair without the usual curves in his back (sway back and hunched shoulders). His whole body, from the top of his head down to his heels, is in good, comfortable alignment.

Now I want to move the student from standing to sitting. It goes like this:

I ask the student to think of his head floating up toward the ceiling, with a slightly forward curve, without making any movement in that direction. The student is also told to think of the back and spine lengthening up toward the ceiling, while the top of the head is leading—something like a kite going up (the head), and the string that is attached to it is lengthening upwards at the same time (the spine).

I stress to Paul that he is to give these thoughts lightly and easily, without moving any muscles, without trying to *do* it in any way, and particularly without going stiff and rigid.

My hands are poised lightly on the back of his head and under his chin. Again, I feel the upward flow in the student's body. To me it is a thrilling moment. I start to move Paul towards the chair, asking him to gradually allow the knees and hip joints to bend and to continue to *think* of his head going forward and up and his back lengthening. He is *thinking upwards* while his body is moving down towards the chair.

As he bends his knees and thinks upwards, I gently guide him. In this way, he experiences the act of sitting down in a chair as being light and airy. He has sat down without the usual throwing of his head backwards and chin up in the air, without hunching his shoulders, without shortening or contracting the back of his neck, without tightly arching the middle of his back, without sticking his buttocks out behind, without straining his thigh muscles.

Not everyone has all of these poor sitting habits. The most common is throwing the head backwards, shortening the neck, and tightening the middle of the back. In the lesson, instead of going through his or her usual aberrations, the student moves to the chair with the head, neck, back and buttocks in one smooth line, the legs bending freely with the feeling of well-oiled joints.

It doesn't matter whether one is sitting down or standing up, or going in or out of either of these positions. The mental directions are the same—"Neck free, head forward and up, back lengthening and widening"—or, in short, "Think upwards."

It is based on the relationship of the head to the top of the spine, which allows the back and the spine to lengthen.

No other instructions are necessary.

▶ Why the Simplicity of the Alexander Technique Works

This process has been confirmed by Professor George E. Coghill, the eminent American biologist, an admirer of Alexander, who discovered the same law of nature in his laboratory experiments, initially with salamanders and later with other vertebrates.

The fact that the head leads and the spine and the rest of the body follows is basic in nature. He discovered that when he interfered with the head movement of salamanders, the body could not move.*

---

*Appendix II in *The Resurrection of the Body*—"Preface to Book by Alexander" by George E. Coghill.

This can be seen clearly in horses. When riding a horse, and you want to stop, pull the head back, and the horse is forced to stop. When you want the horse to turn to the side, you turn the head in that direction, and his body must follow. It is the same with other animals.

We human beings have a much more highly developed cortical brain than any other species, though it is at the expense of some of the benefits of the lower stem brain. The stem brain controls the simple reflex movements. Young babies are capable of doing only these simple movements. As the baby grows and the cortical brain develops, it becomes capable of performing more complex movements. Human beings are able to perform movements that no animal can do, such as skilled tasks with the hands, and most important, standing upright.

We attain more highly developed thought capacity and more physical skills than any other species. But, as the function of the stem brain diminishes, we start to lose the capacity to do the very first simple reflex movements, especially those that we no longer do in our culture beyond babyhood or childhood. At first, the head leads the body. Then most of us learn to move without the head leading. We walk, sit, stand, bend, reach with the chest sticking out and leading, or the neck is forward and leads, or the belly.

When this happens, the head is thrown backwards and the back of the neck is shortened. Now the body is unable to function at its best. The back of the neck becomes tight. The skin under the chin is stretched abnormally, eventually creating a sagging jawline. Back muscles are shortened and tightened. The muscles that go up and down the front of the torso become flabby from overstretching. Pectoral muscle flabbiness means sagging breasts, abdominal muscle flabbiness means a protruding belly. The shoulders become scrunched—either upwards, downwards, forwards, or backwards—with the result of stiff shoulder joints. The hip and knee joints no longer move as freely as the muscles surrounding them become tight and taut—and stiff.

Usually, we are not aware that we are moving around in an unnatural manner. These abnormal ways of moving, sitting and standing, and the tension in our muscles, creep up on us gradually. We don't usually notice it. In fact, we often don't even feel it.

One day, we look in the mirror and see a sway back, rounded shoulders, and a neck that sticks way forward, with buttocks that stick way backwards. Our legs are at an angle instead of being dynamic and straight, the feet are either turned out or turned in.

Or, if we don't notice this in the mirror, we find it becomes difficult to find clothes that fit properly. One shoulder doesn't hang correctly. A pant leg is shorter than the other. The right sleeve is longer than the left. There are wrinkles on one side of a blouse or sweater or shirt, or there are wrinkles on both sides. The stripes on a shirt or sweater are crooked or curved instead of straight.

Perhaps we even don't notice these things in our clothes, but do find that we are starting to get a stiff neck or back or tightness across the shoulders, even after standing or sitting in one position for only five minutes. Our leg joints start to creak. We can't bend down as far as we used to or sit upright easily anymore.

It is then that serious physical problems can start to develop.

There may be pain, either constant or ones that come and go— pain in the neck and shoulders, a burning sensation in the upper back between the shoulder blades, or pain in the upper spine. Pain in the lower back can occur, along with sensation down one leg, or both legs, or aching feet, or numbness in a leg or an arm, in a hand or foot.

Some pain can be so bad that it prevents us from moving. A muscle spasm in the back or in the neck—the end-result of constant tension in those muscles—causes the muscles to lock into a tight position. This can happen over some simple movement like turning the head, or bending to pick up a pencil or reaching for the telephone. Suddenly, we cannot unbend again, or turn the head in the other direction. Muscle spasm is the final step on a long road of constant, persistent muscle tension.

And we ask, "Why me?"

Then along comes the Alexander method, and the brain remembers. The muscles respond. The unwanted learning is dropped. The natural way is relearned.

You can almost hear your body say, "That is so good. What took you so long?"

Some people have cried with joy when they first reexperienced the good feeling in their body.

Using the Mind

When we use the mind to direct the organism, we need to be very specific and need to know exactly what it is that we are directing. For that reason, it is important that there be a teacher to assist the student in identifying the sensation of "Neck free, head forward and up, back lengthening and widening."

The student can automatically associate—on a subconscious level, or at the level of the nervous system—the sensation he experiences with the words that are given. In the Alexander lesson, the teacher repeats the words aloud over and over again, while the student is asked to say the words silently. The teacher's hands assist gently. The connection is made between the brain, the nervous system, and the muscles. It is a conditioning process, and at the same time a deconditioning process.

Most people move with too much tension. There is too much unnecessary work going on in their muscles—much more than is required. As soon as a person starts to stand up, or sit down, or move an arm, the movement is done with too much work, too much tension. If the thought of every movement is connected with too much work, then there will *always* be too much work.

By giving yourself the Alexander mental directions, you begin to undo this. Many repetitions of good directions are needed to effect a fruitful change.

In an Alexander lesson, the hands of the teacher sense and feel every response in the body, no matter how minute or subtle. Because of this, the teacher can give instant feedback and guidance, and the student can fully experience the natural sense of moving freely, as the back lengthens and the head floats forwards and upwards. It is a truly joyous sensation.

When giving yourself the thoughts on your own, without a teacher, you can get a taste of that sensation. When you have the teacher to guide you and to help you go further than you can go on your own, then you come closer to reaching your fullest capacity of good functioning. Alexander called this good "use." Even in the first lesson with a teacher, you can reach a greater degree of improvement than you could on your own.

Patrick Macdonald, one of the foremost Alexander teachers of our day, has expressed our condition in his own words, in his article "The Alexander Technique—Psycho-Physical Integrity":

> "It is possible to demonstrate two forces, or sets of forces, acting in the human body, and, in particular, along the spine . . . They may possibly have something in common with the Positive and Negative of Western science or the Chinese Yin and Yang. Force 'A' has a tendency to contract and distort. It is closely allied to the pull of gravity and causes a 'heaviness' in the body which is not the heaviness of avoirdupois. Force 'B' has an expansionary or elongatory tendency. It is often referred to in a general way, as 'life.' It produces a 'lightness' in the body, which I take to be the natural . . . condition. This lightness . . . has an antigravitational direction . . . It is necessary, therefore, in order to bring the body back to a state of integrity, to minimize the effect of force 'A' and restore that of 'B'. This, though a fairly simple piece of reeducation, is subtle and needs the help of a highly skilled teacher."

I have talked about sitting down and standing up. These two activities are essential in our daily life, and are both involved with the gravitational force. We work largely with the activities of sitting and standing in an Alexander lesson, and we include many other activities.

Sitting in our society involves something not all societies have. This something is the cause of many of our problems.

▶ What the Chairs You Sit in Do to You

Chairs are not natural. They were invented long after man evolved. Man used to squat on the ground, and chairs are still not used in some societies. In our sophisticated Western civilization and in those that have imitated us, chairs are a way of life.

Alexander referred to the chair as "the worst instrument of our civilization." He saw chairs doing so much harm to the human body. He saw them cause stiffness and tension in the hip joints, shortening the leg muscles, decreasing the agility of the knee joints, pulling down the lower back and bringing too much compression into the spine, and shortening and tightening the back of the neck, which in turn pulls the head backwards and downwards.

As a result of slumping in chairs, being upright at any time became more difficult for the human body. Since he saw that we are not going to turn back the clock and do away with the chair, he directed himself to teaching people how to get onto a chair with good, natural alignment, how to maintain that while sitting on a chair, and how to get out of a chair with the muscles moving naturally.

Note: The sitting positions shown on pages 30 and 31 are positions that allow the leg muscles to remain lengthened, and allow the hip joints to remain open and free; in contrast, sitting on a chair does not lengthen the leg muscles, and the hip joints do not remain as open.

I would like to quote Judith Leibowitz in her article "For the Victims of our Culture: THE ALEXANDER TECHNIQUE"*:

"... hundreds of variations upon the shape of the chair have been produced, many differing enormously in terms of how one must sit in them. Indeed, WE, not the chair, have made the compromise. We have agreed to adjust our bodies to the dictates of chairs; only rarely do we find a chair that in its design has contracted to fulfill the requirements of the human body. In such ways have we pemitted the forms and products of our

*Dance Scope Fall, 1969, Vol. 4 Number 1

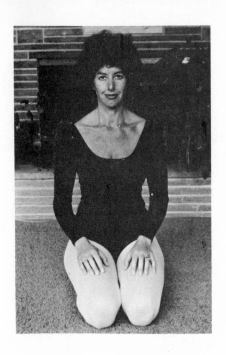
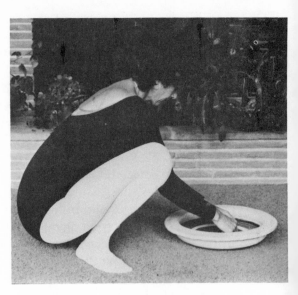

culture to change our body alignments in order to satisfy THEIR structural requirements. We have accustomed ourselves to habitual modes of use that are literally disfiguring. Alexander felt that man must now catch up with his culture, and the way to do that is to learn (or relearn) consciously the proper use of his body. The mechanisms for this use exist in our bodies . . ."

When we sit down, we are going down *with* gravity, and when we are standing up, we are going up *against* gravity. When a body is accustomed to moving in a poor way, involving tension and poor posture of one kind or another, the muscles are not doing their job properly and they give in to gravity. Then we slump down with gravity, or we make an enormous stressful effort to stay up against it.

When we learn to move up to standing—which is going against gravity—with all our muscles and limbs moving with ease, and when we learn to go down onto a chair—which is going down with the pull of gravity—without being pulled down into a slump or hunching up our shoulders against the pull of gravity, then we are capable of performing every movement of daily life with ease.

To continue quoting Patrick Macdonald from his article "The Alexander Technique—Psycho-Physical Integrity":

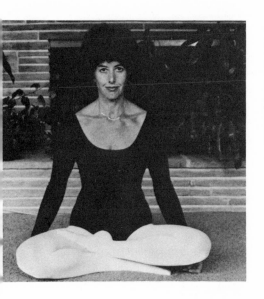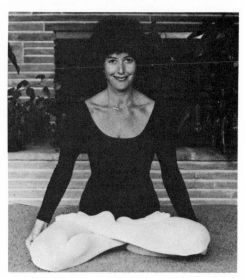

"... an individual orientation of the body, in space, is an essential if the progressive deterioration of man is to be arrested. His thinking about a very large number of other things will have to be reoriented as well. He will have to learn not to ask mythical questions such as 'How should I hold my head and spine?' and learn to ask real ones, as, 'How should my head and spine hold me?' Not 'What position should I sit in?' but 'How can I use myself best in a sitting position?' "

Sitting down and standing up are the two movements we do that are involved with gravity in a major way. In comparison, bending down or reaching up with the arms are a minor involvement.

Of course, a dancer, or an acrobat or a gymnast has other far more difficult movements to do. These people, too, can improve their performances, and perform their arts with far greater ease, greater accomplishment and less practice, when their bodies are functioning at their best in their daily lives. When the body is not functioning efficiently in such daily life actions as sitting and standing, the performer has to work extra hard and put far more strain into performing well in other physical acts. That in itself reduces the quality and the degree of the performance, and requires far more practice, and burns out the body, and the talent, far sooner than necessary. I have observed that performers, artists, and athletes who continue to be great as they grow older, have very good use, for example, Margot Fonteyn, Artur Rubinstein, the late Richard Tucker, David Oistrakh, and Andrés Segovia.

▶ Scientific Evidence of Mind/Body Connection

You may be asking by now "How can muscles change when you are only using thoughts, and not moving your muscles?"

Several years ago, a scientific experiment was reported in *Newsweek*:

> A subject on a chair had the electrodes of an electromyograph attached to his right arm. (An electromyograph is a machine that records muscular movement.) The subject was asked to think of moving his right arm, but to *not* make any movement. When the subject thought of moving his right arm, the electromyograph recorded muscular movement. The subject was certain that he had not moved a muscle, and the researchers had observed no movement in the subject's arm. Several experiments along these lines were made, all showing evidence that the *thought* of a movement brought about muscular movement, although the movement was too slight to be observable.

A well-trained Alexander teacher can see these slight movements, and, eventually, so do some of the students. With the increase in their sensitivity/awareness people can see and observe things that they were blind to before.

Now try an experiment for yourself. Walk around the room. Stop. Walk around the room again, this time pretending that the room is full of unfriendly people. Stop. Walk around the room again and pretend that the room is full of friendly people. Did you feel changes in the degree of tension in your body, changes in your musculature? Did the thought of unfriendly people make your muscles tighten, and did the thought of friendly people make your muscles relax and bring more freedom to your walk? Now you have experienced for yourself how thoughts can affect muscles.

➡️ The People Who Learn the Technique
And How They Benefit

A prominent economist, who held a prestigious position with a major oil company, came to me for Alexander lessons. He was in agonizing pain from a disc problem in the spine. Every day he wore a supportive corset which relieved him from pain sufficiently so that he could go to work and do his job. As soon as he removed his corset, he was in such pain he was unable to function. His doctors told him the only recourse would be a risky back operation that could possibly leave him crippled or paralyzed.

For ten years, he had suffered from back pain. The Alexander Technique had been recommended to him by his friends, and he always put them off. Now, in desperation, he came for lessons to avoid the operation. I insisted that he come three times a week, which he did. He came early in the morning before going to his office. He took off his corset and we began. Within the first month, he was going for longer and longer periods of time without his corset, pain-free. After one month, he had his monthly checkup with his physician. Until then, each month, the physician had pronounced him worse than before. This time, the physician said he was no worse and no better.

He continued his lessons. Despite the fact that both his physician and I stressed that he should do no physical activity outside of his job and that he should rest a lot, he would frequently go sailing on weekends, haul in wood for the fireplace, and play actively with his little girl. He was in more pain when he came for his Monday lesson. However, there was a steady gradual progress, and eventually he had no pain at any time, regardless of whatever physical activity he did.

After the second month, his doctor said he had improved. After three months his doctor pronounced him cured. He continued his lessons with me for some time, until I moved from New York to California.

Five years later, I had a call from him telling me that he was going to be in Los Angeles on business and would like to take a lesson from me again. I learned from him that even though he had not continued his lessons after I left New York, he had never had any pain in his back again, not even a twinge.

My dress designer student told me early one summer about her niece who was on vacation from college and was staying with her family in New York for the summer. The niece was a social failure: fat, morose, withdrawn, hostile and resentful. She refused to listen to any suggestions from her family or friends. However, when her famous aunt suggested the Alexander lessons to her, she agreed to go. Two months later, she had lost 25 pounds, felt radiant, became outgoing, and a social success. She looked forward to going back to school to start a new life.

A tall young woman, who could have been attractive, but looked dowdy and uninteresting, came for lessons to improve her posture. After each lesson, she would look at herself in the large mirror in my studio. After a short while she was able to recognize changes that occurred in her posture.

One day, while taking stock of herself in the mirror at the end of the lesson, she said to me, "You know, when I put on my clothes in the morning they look fine to me, but lately, when I look at myself in the mirror after the lesson, my clothes look dowdy." The next time I saw her, she had changed the style of clothes she was wearing. They now fitted her new alive, joyous appearance. She later started to use make-up and taking better care of her hair. She became an almost transformed creature, attractive, with a joyous happiness radiating from her.

A young medical doctor came for lessons out of curiosity. After only a month of sessions his posture was erect and vital, his face more alive and less strained. The most remarkable benefit to him was that he no longer felt fatigued. He explained that he worked on his feet all day long, and each day he used to feel so tired he could barely stay up. Now he went through the day comfortably, giving better attention to his patients.

A young man who had the position of librarian at a large university came to take lessons after having been impressed by a demonstration of the work. He was a very serious, rather severe young man, with very little expression on his face and a great deal of rigidity in his body. As the lessons progressed, his face became softer, glowing, and more full of expression. His body became light and fluid. His personality became more open and expansive. One day he said to me, "I've noticed that my personality has changed and my attitude at the library has changed. I used to take every little thing very seriously, just as the other librarians do, and now I observe that a lot of things that they take so seriously are unimportant. I realize that I used to be like them and I am happy I am not anymore." Soon after, he applied to be trained as a teacher and was accepted in one of the Alexander training schools.

A nine-year-old boy was brought for lessons three times a week by his mother. He was very slow, awkward, and uncoordinated in his movements and was the laughingstock of his class. He looked unhappy. Luckily, children respond even faster than adults do. The improvement in the boy's coordination was clearly obvious from one lesson to another and his face displayed more aliveness and alertness.

In the third week, his mother reported he had received an "A" in spelling for the first time. The following week, she told me he was getting "A's" in everything. She explained that when he first started school, he had been a brilliant child, then in the third grade he had started to deteriorate and did not do well at school at all. Now after three weeks of Alexander lessons, he was alert, well-coordinated, and functioning at his best again.

A 59-year-old lady came for lessons after reading the April 1967 article in *Harper's Bazaar* about the Alexander Technique, entitled "Take Inches Off Your Waist." She came to get rid of her "spare tire" around her waist.

In the process she reported that her feet no longer ached, and she could play golf for longer periods and more frequently during the week; she had less fatigue altogether; she lost 11 pounds as she found she could stay on a diet easily since she had better feelings in her

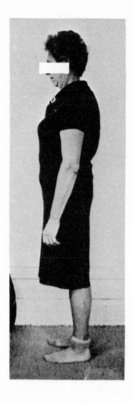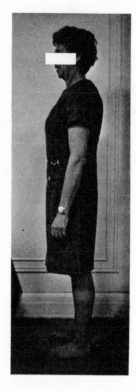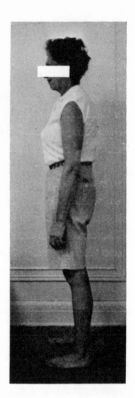

body; and, to her delight, she lost her double chin and her dowager's hump together with her spare tire.

These are dramatic cases. Oftentimes the results do not involve the loss of unwanted weight, improved grades, greater progress at work. Instead, the results are less obvious, but just as welcome.

There is one consistent result: joy, and an improvement in the quality of life.

And that is the real story of the Alexander Technique, a way to free the body and free the mind. It is a way to a new life, with dramatic discoveries about yourself, your experiences, and your peak fulfillment.

The Alexander Technique is a way of life.

Come with me now along that way.

Chapter 2

Free the Body— Free the Person

I Feel As If My Body Is Out of Prison

PEOPLE ARE BORN with freedom of the body, a beauty of body, mind and spirit.

We gradually become prisoners of our tensions, emotional and physical.

When the personality becomes warped, the body becomes warped, and when the body becomes warped, the personality becomes warped.

We respond in our own unique way to our own special stresses. It can start at a very early age. A frightened child and a child in a respressive family and culture already starts to be warped in body and mind. We have separated ourselves from our source of goodness in order to cope with survival in a difficult world and in the process we have isolated ourselves from each other. With each separation we are further removed from goodness and oneness, and more exposed to the buffeting encountered in the war for individual survival. We have wounds old and new. We are bent from the burdens we carry. We are weary and in need of relief.

The intertwining of body and personality is eloquently expressed by Ron Kurtz and Hector Prestera, M.D.:*

The Body Reveals—An Illustrated Guide to the Psychology of the Body (Harper and Row)

"The body never lies. Its tone, color, posture, proportions, movements, tensions, and vitality express the person within . . . The body says things about one's emotional history and deepest feelings, one's character and personality . . .

"It is often easy to recognize a person by his walk . . . In doing so, we use the same cues that tell us of his life-style. A drooping head, slumped shoulders, a caved-in chest, and a slow, burdened gait reflect feelings of weakness and defeat, while a head carried erect, shoulders straight and loose, a chest breathing fully and easily, and a light gait tell of energy and confident promise . . .

"*Fixed muscular patterns in the body are central to a person's way of being in the world* . . . (italics are mine)

" . . . It is as if the body sees what the mind believes and the heart feels, and adjusts itself accordingly. This gives rise to a way of holding oneself, as pride can swell the chest or fear contract the shoulders . . .

"Ideally, the body is capable of allowing the free flowing of any feeling. It is efficient and graceful in its movements, aware and responsive . . . Such a body has bright eyes, breathes freely, is smooth skinned, and *has an elastic muscle tone. It is well proportioned . . . The neck is pliable and the head moves easily . . . The entire body is lined up efficiently with respect to gravity . . .* (italics are mine) Pleasure and well-being are the characteristic feelings. A person with such a body is emotionally flexible and his or her feelings are spontaneous."

When that relief comes, can you imagine your joy? In a word, one could call it a relief from *stress*.

Symposia on stress are now commonplace. These are one or two day events and are usually conducted by physicians, psychologists, nurses and other health care professionals. These are the people who must deal with the consequences of stress on people. They must help people identify the causes of stress and manage its levels. Such symposia are usually quite thorough in their intellectual analyses of the subject, the way stress affects the mind and body, and methods for adapting to it. Behavior therapy is often introduced as a means of countering maladaptive stress responses. But what about the wounds and warps already suffered? What about you and I, here and now? What can we do to restore ourselves? What can we do to be free of the scars of stress that threaten to cloud our happiness, interfere with our productive skills, and shorten our lives?

▶ Enter Joy of Body, Mind and Spirit

When your body is freed of the effects of repeated past stress, it literally breathes a sigh of relief. Vital organs and systems function normally once again. Life energy surges in restored abundance.

When the mind is freed of the stressed body, it too breathes a sigh of relief. It has been making a subliminal accommodation to tensed ligaments, distorted internal spaces, a disrupted nervous system and impeded functioning. Release from that "prison" brings a sense of euphoria as the life energy is released to give you a lifelong "high," and brain neurons are freed to resume their contributions to total intelligence. An unseen ballast has been removed. Your spirit soars. Your life begins to have more meaning. You have more compassion and understanding, more sensitivity to yourself and others. You are more able to give and to receive love. You no longer feel as separate and alone. Stress dissolves. Without stress—competition, anxiety, insecurity, hostility and the like—we are more together. This to-getherness is on a person-to-person basis, and simultaneously on a universal plane. We feel more "in tune" with nature. We restore our wholeness with society and the world.

At the moment this might sound almost alien to you. However, as you do some of the simple stress-releasing activities on the pages ahead you will understand the promise of the Alexander Technique. When you have a tension headache, you do not appreciate the fact that the sky is blue and the weather balmy. When you have a gnawing backache, you are not aware of your blessings. Even if the effects of stress are not shouting at you through pain, you are still virtually blindfolded to the fullest joys that life can bring. At this moment it is a fairy tale concept. "Maybe for them, but not for me."

Not so.

It is for you. You are part of the human "family." And though such joy may be beyond your reach and belief now, expect a change.

▶ The Many Levels of Separation

We like to be alone in our misery. The quiet desperation that the struggle for survival entails is a fracturing force. It separates the strugglers from each other and from their own natures. This emotional separation produces its counterpart in the body. It, too, becomes separated in a way. It is no longer integrated and may indeed disintegrate. There is also, apparently, a non-integrated aspect to body, mind and spirit. Such a person is mentally out of touch with the body and even "lost" in spirit. When this person takes steps to restore this separation of his or her three-fold nature, a balancing takes place. Another indication of this lack of integration is

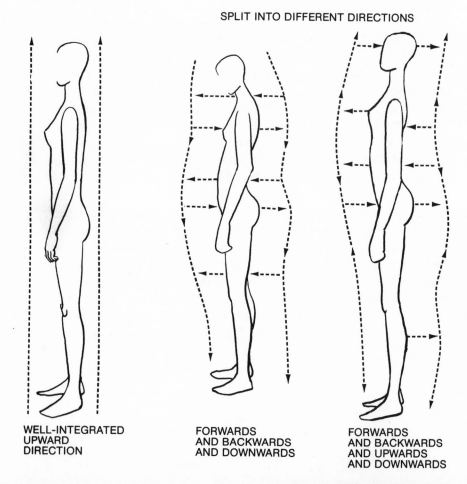

SPLIT INTO DIFFERENT DIRECTIONS

WELL-INTEGRATED
UPWARD
DIRECTION

FORWARDS
AND BACKWARDS
AND DOWNWARDS

FORWARDS
AND BACKWARDS
AND UPWARDS
AND DOWNWARDS

the way the body holds together. There seem to be a lot of ill-fitting parts. The legs seem to be reluctant to follow the torso, the stomach wants to steal the show, or the arms and hands don't seem to know what to do, as if they had just arrived on the scene and don't belong.

The personality of people fractured by stress seems separated. They are of one mood one day or one minute, another mood the next. They are unpredictable. If you are such a person, you have your good days and your bad days. You might also be contradictory. As a parent, you might say yes to the child today, and no tomorrow for the same request, causing stress to others. So it is that fractured-by-stress people add to the stress of the environment, dividing and conquering, splitting and shattering body, mind, and spirit. Perhaps the essence of Alexander's contribution to humanity is that by normalizing one area of stress—the body—you can trigger an integration of the whole person, and by inference, of society. The body parts begin to fit together and function as a more harmonious whole. The person "gets his head together" and the personality emerges into a unique and pleasing focus. Such a person gets along better with family, neighbors, friends and co-workers. There is a oneness with society, other life-styles, and cultures. There is a unity with nature. There is a unity with mankind. Just as a loss of a job, or an illness in the family can trigger a fracturing chain reaction, so can a body-mind balance in the Alexander way trigger an integrating chain reaction. Your universe is put back together again. You are transformed.

➡ The Burdens of The World Are on Your Shoulders

When a person says, "It changed my life," what does that person really mean? When a person goes from a state of confusion to a state of euphoria, what is really happening inside?

I used to feel the stress of survival acutely. I felt that the burdens of the world were all mine, and my shoulders showed it. They were stooped. I was not only droopy and round-shouldered, I was also sway-backed.

One day, as I was walking home after one of my Alexander lessons, I was thinking of some problems I had. They were the same problems that had burdened me in the past before I started my Alexander lessons. They were the same problems that had stooped my shoulders and swayed my back, and made me feel heavy and depressed. But now, as I walked along the sidewalk with these problems, I felt a difference. They did not seem to bear down on me. In fact, they seemed to be floating in the air above my head, several inches away from my body. Even though I still had these weighty problems, my body felt light, and upright, and bouncy. The fact that I had problems to think about did not interfere with the vital and alive feeling

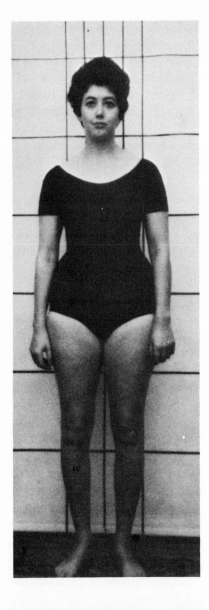 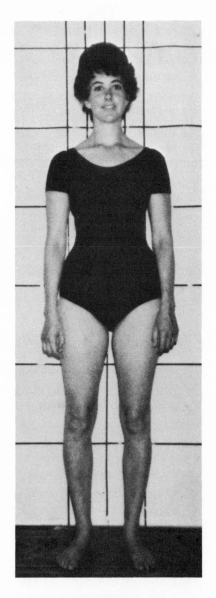

that my body had derived from the Alexander lesson. I walked with a spring in my step under the same circumstances in my life that only weeks before had warped my body. I also walked without a mental or emotional burden. The answers to my problems came to me, easily. I acted on these answers optimistically. I was able to address the problems eagerly.

I no longer feel that the burdens of the world are mine. I still have

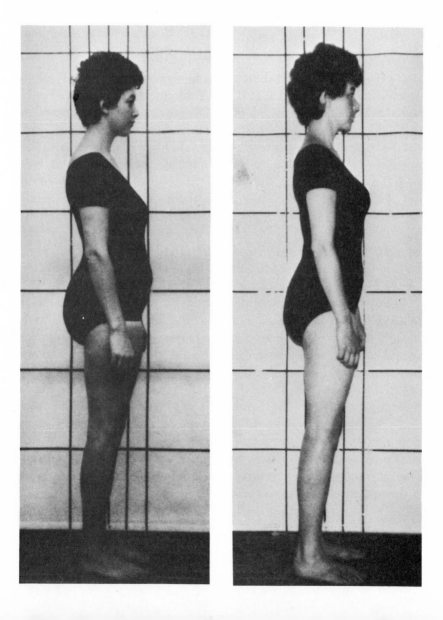

my ups and downs but the ups are higher and the downs are less pronounced. I found out that day that the burdens of the world had been sitting on my shoulders and what joy it was to let them be disconnected and float away from my body. Even today, when I have problems and mention to my friends that I do, my friends express surprise. They say I look vital and alive, as if I did not have a care in the world. I see this in my students, too. Apparently, removing the signs of stress from the body has a lasting effect. It enhances and protects. It seems to disconnect the circuitry that makes weighty problems signal their physical counterparts.

▶ What It Means to "Change Your Life"

I used to feel that I didn't want to continue to live . . . I was so unhappy with myself. I find it incredible today to think this could have been me. Today my "depths of despair" are highs compared to those days. And my capacity for joy is multiplied many times over. My body responds most readily with joy. I feel it all the way to the marrow of my bones. Circumstances outside the body respond, too. I used to have very few friends. My friends were people who used me. I used to feel very inferior to them. They were my friends because I did things for them, and they would not do anything for me. Today, people like me for my own sake. My friends are real friends. Some of them are the same friends as before, others are new. I no longer feel inferior to others. I feel a strength in myself that comes together with the changes in my body.

Before I took the Alexander lessons, I was a droopy, gloomy-looking person. I attracted spineless "leeches." I was a social wall-flower. At a party, if a man came up to me and danced with me, he would soon excuse himself. The only ones that stayed around were lost souls or what we girls called "drips." The attractive guys never seemed to look at me. Those that did, didn't stay around more than a few minutes. In my "after" picture, you see me more upright, erect and vibrant. I attracted a different type of person that "goes" with that nature—attractive people . . . people who were attractive in personality and often also in their looks. As the people in your life change, circumstances change. It becomes a cycle that feeds itself. It is the opposite of a vicious cycle. It is a joyous cycle.

After I had a significant number of Alexander lessons, I found that at parties attractive men flocked around me . . . and attractive women, too. People wanted to develop friendships with me—it happens everywhere I go. For many years now, instead of being able to count my friends on one hand, I need to discriminate and choose among those who wish to be close to me. My love life, my social life, my economic life were transformed. This is the story of my life: the one-time ugly duckling wallflower—transformed by the Alexander Technique. These changes are not unique to me. They happen to other Alexander students. They can happen to you.

Alexander students who are in therapy—either psychotherapy or physical therapy—report that they have breakthroughs in their therapy when they start their lessons, and their therapists also remark on the sudden progress.

Whenever somebody says to me, "The lessons have changed my life," I know exactly what they mean.

➡ Why Changes For the Better Occur In Your Sex Life

You will be going through some mind-body experiences with me from time to time as you progress through the book. They will produce changes that you can notice and which will give you a taste of joy, a taste of the banquet ahead. Blocks and armorings are relinquished. Openness and receptivity take their place. You join "with" whatever you are doing. I used to be a person who couldn't participate when others were being witty and humorous, or when people were being fun-loving and playful. I stood apart feeling as if I were a block of wood. I deeply envied those who were witty, and longed to be like them. Those who were being playful, I thought of as silly and childish and I felt superior to them. Does that sound familiar to you—to feel both inferior and superior? "Split" in how we feel is connected with a "split" in the body—that is, one part of the body is different than another part—one part is weak, another strong; one part flexible, another stiff; one part tight, another flabby. A body of "ill-fitting" parts—instead of a beautifully integrated, harmonious, supple body, with all the parts flowing smoothly.

The "new" me is a person who participates easily in witty and humorous situations and joyfully in fun-loving play, who harmonizes and flows with others, instead of standing apart. I enjoy everything more—dancing, walking, sports, music, sex, being with people. Many others have found the same.

Arthur, a psychologist, came to me for lessons because of a painful back. He was in his fifties, and he walked stiffly. He was quiet and reserved. Even his face was rigid. After the third lesson, a change came over his face. It was as if he had taken off a mask. His face became alive, more vital. His body followed. The back pain lessened, and soon disappeared altogether. A calisthenics enthusiast, he was able to resume exercises which he had had to avoid because of his back problem. As his body became more flexible, his whole demeanor softened. One day after an Alexander lesson, Arthur was telling me of the improvements he was experiencing. "You know, something else has happened. I last longer in the sexual act." He told me he had been divorced for some time and that his marital difficulties were at least partially due to the problem of "finishing" too soon. The problem remained, though, after his divorce and was inhibiting his new relationships. He was seeking a marriage partner and now he felt a serious block had been removed.

What was the cause-effect relationship here? Of course, the back was an important factor. A painful back made it imperative that Arthur get the sex act over with as quickly as possible. But even if pain were not a factor, Arthur could not control his sexual pleasure with arigid back as well as he could once his back became more flexible. A rigid back means a rigid pelvis, a flexible back allows the pelvis to be flexible. The controls came about naturally and pleasurably.

In reviewing Arthur's case, I am reminded of my own. My first love relationship was a beautiful and exciting sexual experience. However, I never experienced an orgasm. My lover was very skilled, and I often felt close to coming through but it never happened. Years went by, and I had the capacity to enjoy sex—usually feeling quite satisfied from the good feelings involved, and at other times feeling frustrated. Then one time it happened. My partner had done nothing different. But I had. I had taken Alexander lessons. Later, after teaching for a few years and seeing the changes in my students and connecting them with the sexual improvements they reported, I understood more clearly what had happened. To function fully and freely, the pelvis needs to be free. Inadequate functioning can take different forms. For me, it was inability to achieve orgasm. As my pelvis became freed in the Alexander lessons, I moved more freely in sexual activity. The backward tilt of the pelvis due to my sway back disappeared. My pelvis fell into good alignment and allowed the stream of sexuality to flow unhindered to completion.

Sandra was another example. She came from a moralistic home. Sex was frowned on, especially for a woman. Married in her early twenties, Sandra brought her Victorian attitude toward sex with her on the honeymoon. The result was anything but good. She participated reluctantly. She could not "surrender" to her husband in the act of love.

The Alexander lessons brought Sandra more in touch with her own body. She became softer, more open. The more this happened, the more she invited it to happen in her physical activities, including sex. As she became more open in the act of love, she was able to let down her defenses and surrender to her husband. It made all the difference between an act of duty and an act of ecstasy.

Lorna, a green-eyed photographer's model, lived in an elegant apartment with her executive husband. They had been married five years. Lorna had a good figure, although she had a flat chest and flat, turned-under buttocks. She came for Alexander lessons for an apparently minor reason: one shoulder was slightly lower than the other. The designer for whom she modeled had taken Alexander lessons from me and told her, "I don't want to be always adjusting my clothes for you. Take Alexander lessons. Get your shoulders leveled out." After a few lessons, her shoulders evened out. But that was not all. She developed pleasingly rounded buttocks, and her bust looked fuller. "My husband says I look more sexy," she said as she looked at herself in my studio's full-length mirror. Two weeks later she added, "My husband says I not only look more sexy, I *am* more sexy." She turned to me with a beaming smile and said, "He thinks he brought about the changes, but I know better. I know it was Alexander. But I let him think it was him!"

Although I have attributed sexual changes for the better to improved pelvic and back flexibility and improved breathing, this is an over-simplification. There is a deeper body-mind-spirit change. You can see it in the glow and radiance of Alexander students. The change affects far more than muscle and bone. With the Alexander Technique transformations are of the whole person.

Betty, a former model, was another case in point. She was married, with a 9-year-old child. She came for Alexander lessons because of migraine headaches. Her twice-weekly visits brought a progression of comments from her. "My headaches are less intense and do not last as long." "I had one very brief headache." "This week I had no headache." "I don't have migraines any more." "I have been having dreams about my body. I have never had such dreams before." "I like the way my body feels now." "I enjoy my body. I have never enjoyed it before. I feel more like a female." "I am enjoying sex now. I have never before enjoyed it very much." "My husband is so thrilled that I am enjoying sex for the first time in the ten years of our marriage, he wants me to take five lessons a week!"

Stanley, about 35, was a sturdy, strapping, good-looking man, an engineer. He held his chest out as if his looks depended on it. His chest seemed to call on this teacher's attention for another reason. Its rigidity could be softened. One day, I used some simple breathing techniques during the lesson, together with Alexander directions. While he was lying on the table, with knees bent, I asked him to fill his chest with air and let the air out three or four times; then I asked him to do the same with his belly, then to alternate belly and chest. After just a few minutes of breathing like this, while directing, his chest visibly softened. He seemed a gentler person without any loss of masculinity. He felt the difference himself but his verbalization of it was a surprise. "Judith, I feel so warm towards you. You're an attractive woman and I've wanted to have sex with you since I met you. But now I don't feel that. I feel tender and warm towards you."

The "techniques" are so gentle and so simple. Many find it hard to believe that so much can happen with so little. And how fast these releases can come!

Bones, muscles, and nerves are quick to respond, but who would think that the skin could be affected? Mildred, 14, was a bright girl, with a cramped body and a shy manner and bad skin. She was small and thin for her age and could not look me in the eye. She seemed to be intimidated by life. Her mother was an excessively lively, dominant person. I was embarrassed for Mildred at the way her mother treated her, with a total lack of sensitivity and disregard for Mildred's feelings. No wonder she was intimidated! As the lessons progressed, the child's attitude changed. A straighter body seemed to free something within her. She talked more readily with me. Her shyness gave way to radiance. And, to my surprise, her skin cleared up. Acne vulgaris, as its scientific name implies, is a curse to young people. Contrary to what many people think, it is not aggravated by chocolate nor is it improved with soap and water. It is due to oil production caused by the male sex hormone testosterone which is present in males and females. It starts with blackheads and ends with pocks and scars. Dr. Norman Goldstein, a dermatologist and author of *The Skin You Live In*, states that stress is a primary cause of acne. He calls acne sufferers "the most insecure people on earth, socially, sexually, and economically." Usually, a reduction in emotional load causes an improvement in the condition. "Mother can be an emotional load to a child seeking to be its own person," he states. This appeared to be right on target for Mildred. The Alexander lessons freed the resistances to parental stress that she had collected throughout her frail body. She became her own person, and it was not a person with acne.

In Alexander teaching there is emphasis on the body, albeit through the mind. The effects are at first most obvious in the body, then an extension of the joyous effects spreads to mind and spirit, and emotional well-being. The joy in the life of the body is reflected in one's whole being.

➡ The Real Meaning of "Let The Neck Be Free"

When you eavesdropped on an Alexander lesson in the previous chapter, you heard the teacher repeat over and over, "Let the neck be free, to let the head go forward and up, to let the back lengthen and widen." Mentally followed by the student, as simple movements are undertaken physically under the supervision of the teacher, the words have contributed to such widespread effects as better sex, cessation of migraine headaches, and a clear complexion and positive attitude. How is this possible? Let us examine those words more closely.

The first word is "let." This might be the most important word of all. There is no "letting" in stress. If you could "let" in a stressful situation, there would be no stress. There would be a letting go of stress. "Let" the neck be free also avoids a trying or an effort. The effort to *make* the neck free would stiffen the neck, it would reinforce the stress that is already stored in the neck. The concept of "let" comes slowly to students in the first lesson. They tend to try to "make" the neck be free and go through strange contortions to accomplish this. "Letting" it happen is the key. It releases the neck. The neck becomes naturally free. "Letting" means *not* doing anything, *only* directing with your mind, *only* saying the words. Notice also the word "to." It does not stop at the neck. The neck is only the beginning. There is more "letting."

The head is the beneficiary of the next "letting." The neck is freed *to let* the head go forward and up. Here again, a muscular effort to *make* the head go forward and up is directly contrary to what is needed. What is needed is that same permissive letting. In addition to the words, a clear mental image of the head going forward and up is very helpful. (See p. 16.) The concept of having the head go forward and up was seen by Alexander as the opposite of what people were doing wrong. So, it is not meant to be something to "do," rather, something to be "undone." That something is head backwards and downwards (see page 16). "Head forward and up" is an antidote to head backwards and downwards. The change takes place as the antidote takes effect. "Forward" unlocks the head at the atlanto-occipital joint. "Up" permits a slight extension of the spine following this unlocking. For badly slumped individuals this extension of the spine can be quite dramatic, adding an inch or more to a student's height.

"To" and "let" are repeated in the back-directed phase, in order that this be a continuous rather than separated activity, and in order that the back is not *made* to do anything but merely *permitted* to attain its full length and its normal width.

"Let the neck be free" is the key that unlocks the gates. Without that, the head cannot go forward and up, and when the head cannot go forward and up, the spine cannot lengthen. However, neck free, head forward and up, and back lengthening and widening *all happen at once*, simultaneously. They are *not* to be thought of as happening one after the other. This is very important. We are unable to say three phrases all at once, we have no choice but to say them one after the other. In our mind, though, we can have the mental concept of it all happening at the same time.

Alexander was known to express this as: *"All together, one after the other!"*

Your mental concept needs to be accurate, then the words will do the job you want them to do. The meaning of the words and the concepts they represent, are not a "doing" but lead to an "undoing." As the tense parts are released, unnatural stress dissolves. The body returns to its natural balance.

Some people come for Alexander lessons for postural changes. But other changes are inevitable. Carolyn did not believe that anything could change her slumped posture. She had come to accept herself as a slumped, bent-over person. She was negative and depressed-looking and her face had a dragged-down look. In her late forties, she had fundamentally attractive features and the basic ingredients of a good figure but she did not consider herself attractive. She came to the lessons with great skepticism, which she openly expressed. Her skeptical attitude persisted during her first lessons, even though I pointed out improvements to her as we went along. On the fifth lesson she smiled. I had never seen her smile before. From this moment on she became more enthusiastic about the lessons. Still, when I said to her, "You know, Carolyn, your figure has improved," she replied, "I don't really see any change." It was not until several weeks later that this answer changed. "On my way here, a man whistled at me," she beamed. "That has not happened to me in fifteen years. Now I *know* I've changed!" From then on, her skepticism vanished and she became an ardent enthusiast of the lessons and what they were doing for her. She then sent her 10-year-old daughter for lessons and was delighted with the results. Her awkward ten-year old became transformed in a few weeks into a supple, graceful gymnast.

▶ A Simple Exercise to Free the Neck

When you release tension in the neck muscles, they are going to become more lengthened, as a result of less contraction. Here is a very gentle exercise to help release tension in the neck.

Lie down on the floor with your knees bent and your legs and feet spread comfortably apart. Gently roll your head from side to side, left and right, easily and softly. See how it feels. Does it roll smoothly or does it jerk? Is it a gentle, easy movement or does it feel a little difficult? I am going to suggest different ways of doing this.

Leave your head in the middle and look softly at the ceiling. Choose a spot on the ceiling above you to look at. If there is no spot there, imagine that there is a spot. When you look at the spot, please do not stare at it. Instead, breathe normally and blink your eyes easily the way you normally do. Gently roll your head from side to side while your eyes look softly at the spot on the ceiling above you. Naturally, your head doesn't move as much when you don't move your eyes, and the movement is restricted. Do the movement within the range that is comfortable. After several times, six to eight times, allow your eyes to roll with your head. Has the movement of rolling your head become easier and smoother now than it was originally? Is there a difference in the movement? Now allow your head to rest in the middle.

There are several ways in which to improve a movement and the way you move. Here is another way to improve the way you roll your head. When you roll your head, I would like you to realize that the muscles that are rolling your head are in your neck. When the sensation of rolling your head is easier, then you know that your neck muscles have improved and are functioning better. Roll your head again from side to side, and this time think that it is the tip of your nose that is moving through the air. Your head follows your nose because it is attached to your nose. It has no choice, it has to follow. As you roll your head from side to side, do not think about rolling your head, *instead* think about moving your nose through the air right and left. Does this make the rolling of your head even easier? Now leave your head in the middle. Is there any difference in the way the back of your head meets the floor? Is there perhaps less pressure? Is it a different spot on the back of your head that is making the contact with the floor?

Let us experiment with another variation. Roll your head softly from side to side and see again how it feels. Let your head come to the middle. Now imagine that there is a very long feather attached to the tip of your nose, and that the tip of the feather touches the ceiling. Now let that feather move across the ceiling right and left. As your nose is attached to the feather, your nose has to move with it; as your head is attached to your nose, your head has to move with it also. Watch the tip of your feather softly with your eyes, and your eyes will also move. For a moment, think of how your head is rolling now, and whether there is a different quality to the movement; then think again of the tip of your feather. After a few more times, allow your head to rest in the middle, and let your feather vanish. Do your eyes feel different? Are they seeing things differently now?

Once more, roll your head softly right and left, very simply, and think of this as a relaxation rather than an exercise. Does it roll differently than when you first did it? Leave your head in the middle. Gently roll over to one side, leaving your knees bent, and roll all the way onto your hands and knees; from there slowly come up to standing, and look around you. Does your head feel different? Perhaps it feels light. Perhaps it feels higher up, closer to the ceiling than before. Perhaps your neck feels freer, or longer. Leave your head in the middle and see if you feel some change all the way down your back. Perhaps even your legs feel different. Walk around the room and see if walking feels different than before. As you walk, softly turn your head from side to side, and look at things around the room, and see whether that movement is easier. If you do feel greater ease, a lightening in your body, then I think I can say to you that these sensations are akin to what you would get in the first lesson with an Alexander teacher.

You are experiencing the beginning of what "neck free" can do for you.

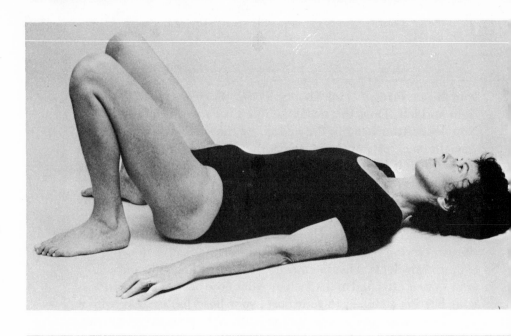

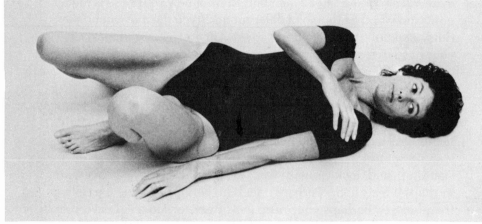

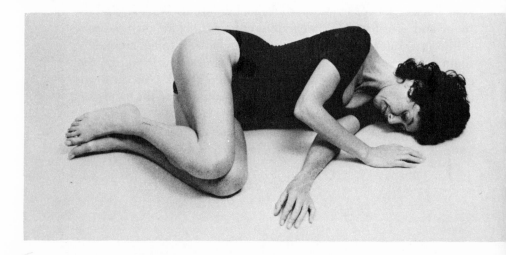

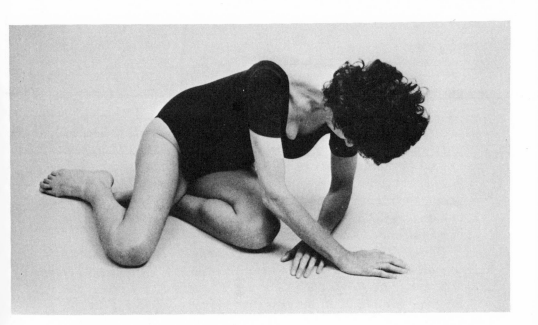

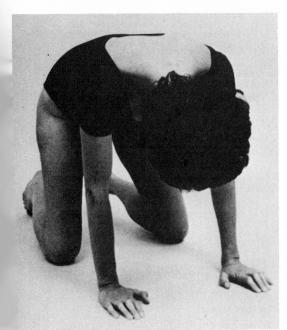

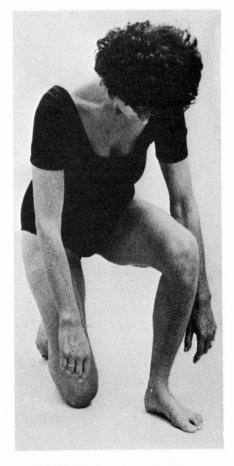

▶ A Freed Neck—More Earning Power?

The body is constantly being affected by the mind. There is no mystery about that. There is a mystery to some people about how the mind can be affected by the body. When Dr. Maxwell Maltz performed cosmetic surgery on habitual criminals, straightening cauliflower ears and correcting pug noses, the rate of their returning to prison after being released was effectively reduced. Apparently the tail can wag the dog. Apparently the body is constantly affecting the mind's attitudes, emotions, and abilities.

There is a *double* feedback system. The brain sends messages to the muscles via the nervous system. For example, your nose itches and you think to yourself, "I'm going to scratch my nose"; the message is transmitted through your nervous system and you lift your hand and scratch your nose. But how did you know that your nose was itching? The sensation in your nose had been transmitted to your mind, via the nervous system, and when the message was received, your mind said "My nose itches." Your mind then sent the message to your hand to scratch your nose.

When the itch is relieved, a message goes to the mind that registers as, "My nose feels fine." The brain then sends a message to the hand to stop scratching the nose.

There are constant messages going in both directions from the brain to the muscles and from the muscles to the brain. A double feedback system.

See if you can sense this for yourself.
1. Stand slumped over, shoulders down.
2. Be aware of your state of mind.
3. Gently straighten up, until you feel natural.
4. Again, be aware of your state of mind.

As you slumped down, did you feel gloomy, and low in spirit? As you straightened up, did your attitude also straighten up? Did you feel less down in the dumps, more optimistic?

This connection between body and mind is affecting the life we live. Its effects are not only the obvious ones we have been examining in this chapter, but they can extend to our functioning in business and in creativity. I have seen Alexander students change jobs. They move from limited jobs to positions with more promise. They move out of locked-in jobs to jobs with more challenge and creativity.

Some people have been unable to work because of severe pain, and felt desperately insecure. In some cases the incapacitating pain was temporary, but occurred again and again, so that those people lived in fear of the next bout, and in fear of having permanent pain and disability—and therefore no income. With Alexander lessons, the pain vanished, sometimes in one week, sometimes in a few weeks—they could resume work with a new joyous spirit. No more fear. As time went by and the pain did not recur, apprehension vanished.

Some people had been limited in their choice of a job because of their pain, and could go on to better things with a renewed self-confidence and enthusiasm.

It is not only the aches and pains that limit people and cause them to lose days of work and efficiency while at work. It goes further and deeper than that. Some of them had no aches and pains to hinder them—there was an inner change that brought them further than before.

No doubt if one attempted to follow the clues, a more direct cause-effect relationship could be delineated. A more comfortable body yields a better disposition which in turn brings a better job. Such an analysis can also take the creativity route. Artists who have taken the Alexander training have experienced dramatic improvements in their work. Dancers, actors, singers, writers, artists, experience new heights of creativity. Of course, here again, the physiological aspect is important, too. The artist does not get tired and strained standing at the easel, a pianist does not get exhausted and tied up in knots, a dancer does not overstrain muscles. In addition, barriers are opened in the body and talent blocks dissolve. Musicians play better. Singers perform better. Dancers dance better. Actors act better. Actors understand immediately the benefits of this psycho-physical bonus, which gives more creativity, productivity, and earning power.

The first people attracted to the Alexander Technique were mostly actors, and later dancers and musicians. A favorite phrase of many actors is, "Free the body, free the voice." Actors of the Tyrone Guthrie Theatre in Minnesota took lessons. It is espoused by William Ball, Director of the American Conservatory Theatre in San Francisco, and recommended by him as essential to every member of the cast no matter how large or small the role. The Alexander Technique is taught in the Drama Department of the Juilliard School in New York. It has been practiced in Shakespearean circles, including the American Festival Theatre in Stratford, Connecticut. All three major Drama Schools in London have Alexander teachers on their staff. The University of Southern California has the Alexander Technique in its Drama Department. The Melbourne Repertory Theater in Australia hires an Alexander teacher for its actors. These are only some of the places where the Alexander Technique is provided for actors. Many major actors of film and stage have privately taken lessons in the Alexander Technique, among them, Joel Grey, Alan Bates, Nina Foch, Joanne Woodward and Paul Newman, Sally Ann Howes, Richard Chamberlain. Some of them say "The Alexander Technique is the best thing I have ever done."

When a person has a certain "set" in his body acquired over years of stress, the body holds itself in a certain posture or alignment. Perhaps the shoulders are held high, or the neck slants forward. An actor with these physical characteristics is cast in roles appropriate to such a set. He is limited in the kinds of roles he can play, dictated by the way his body looks and moves. And because attitude and temperament are linked to body stance, these factors, too, tend to lock the actor into a stereotype.

In their book *The Body Reveals*, Ron Kurtz and Hector Prestera clearly connect the physiology of the body with the psychology of the person. For instance, the person with a rigid body, stiff neck and shoulders and chest held out is frequently someone, they say, with a feeling of being opposed, blocked or challenged. Such a person has difficulty in slowing down. They are sticklers for protocol. They are easily angered.

We commonly associate a strong jaw with determination and aggressiveness, but these authors see in it, too, a holding back of fear and an impulse to cry. We associate a stiffly held neck and shoulders with a singleness of purpose, but seldom realize it also means anger and resentment.

These are the kinds of associations that are undone through the Alexander training. The actor is freed for many roles. The spectrum of creativity is broadened. A physical "set" is replaced by a neutral free state. The body is more pliable. There is more resonance in the voice as vocal chords become more relaxed. Features become more flexible. The actor becomes more versatile.

In the Alexander teaching communication between mind and body is enhanced. As the student visualizes or directs the neck to be free and the head and back to respond, a subconscious effect of mind over body that has been operative over the years is converted into a conscious effect in reverse. A dirt path is converted into a six-lane highway as this communication becomes conscious. Who better than an actor can benefit immediately from this mind-body control?

I am often asked "what if an actor needs to play the role of a rigid person, or an old stooped person?" And I answer "Even if an actor needs to play the role of a hunchback, he hunches over with 'direction,' that means he can direct length even into a stooped posture, and his body does not become as stressed as otherwise in this posture. Then—when his role is over, he can become upright with 'direction,' by giving himself his Alexander Technique directions to erase the contraction of the role and lengthen again upwards."

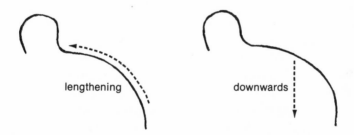

lengthening   downwards

➡ The Intrinsic Energy

The ancient Chinese art of T'ai-chi, though ostensibly a system of flowing movements, is really an exercise in mind-body integration. One must become like a child. One must be relaxed. The head is held as if suspended from the ceiling. The mind concentrates on the top of the head.

Through this mind-body unity, "chi" or intrinsic energy is permitted to flow more freely. Teachers of T'ai-chi find it difficult to explain "chi." We have no word for it in English. In the Alexander Technique we use the word "direction," which I am certain is the same as "chi."

Now, scientists throughout the world are photographing and studying the energy of consciousness and its effects on matter. Perhaps this is the same as "chi." It is this energy which, when modulated with ideas, evolves into creativity. As we experience a new lightness and ease in the movement of our body, we enjoy a more natural health level, fuller flow of mental energy, and a restoration of our spiritual heritage. Our very life energy has been turned on and that warp in the connection has been removed.

I promise you a taste of this joy. I will "take you by the hand" through simple movements that uncrimp your flow of joy. Though not "pure" Alexander, which can only be given in person, these movements will provide a taste of this body-mind awareness. They will give you a body-head start.

It is a great joy for me to be playing a part in this. My joy comes from seeing a concert pianist lose her tenseness and stage fright and speed ahead in her professional career. My joy comes from seeing a shy teenage boy with a pimply face become socially popular and president of the high school class. My joy comes from seeing an average housewife tied to the kitchen sink find a flow of energy and freedom that allows her to take continuing education courses and start new hobbies and interests. My joy comes from seeing an uptight businessman, on the verge of a breakdown, look ten years younger and discover the world outside his financial statements. My joy comes from seeing a person incapacitated by agonizing back pain, or arthritis, become radiant and active again—leading a normal life. My joy will be your joy as we proceed.

A New York actor in his forties, named Michael, came to me for Alexander lessons. It was not for his acting that he came. He had started to learn to play the piano, and he was getting a pain in the neck from sight-reading the music. His piano teacher suggested Alexander. It worked. The tenseness causing the neck pains was averted. And one day, while he was sitting on the chair in the lesson, he suddenly exclaimed, "I feel like a king!" Michael said he had always wanted to feel like a king, but never did. He had played king roles, and had never felt like a king, therefore had never felt natural in the parts. Now he could feel like a king all the time—his dream had come true.

Later, he brought me a specific acting problem. He was rehearsing for a play in which he was required in one scene to walk across the stage toward an actor, intending to beat him up. His director was disturbed over the way he walked, and criticized it as being totally inconsistent with the emotion of the moment. "My director actually crawled on his knees attempting to direct my feet with his hands," Michael explained, "but it did no good, he wasn't satisfied."

He showed me how he walked and I agreed with his director. I asked him to walk across the room saying to himself the Alexander directions—let the neck be free, to let the head go forward and up, to let the back lengthen and widen—and not to try to change his walk in any way.

Then I asked him to repeat this walk, reducing the directions to one word, "lengthen," or "up," and adding the mental thought that he was going to beat up this fellow.

His steady, firm walk brought about by the Alexander directions then acquired a slight overtone to it. It was exactly what the part called for and he reported at the next lesson that his director was satisfied.

We can apply what we learn in the Alexander Technique in many ways—we can give a mental direction for anything we wish—so the Alexander principle of using the mind to direct our behavior is all-encompassing.

Paul Newman, the renowned actor, came for Alexander lessons because of severe backache that prevented him from standing comfortably for even a short period of time. His actress wife, Joanne Woodward, also took lessons.

At the first lesson, while Joanne was watching, I brought Paul up to standing with Alexander direction. He stood there, and after a while he turned to Joanne and said, "I could stand like this for half an hour." He continued to stand there, then he said to her, "I could stand like this for two hours."

And there was joy in his voice.

The layman may not have perceived any difference in the way Paul Newman was standing when he started the lesson and the way he was standing now with no back strain. The difference is often subtle in appearance but not subtle at all in the depth of its effect.

The Alexander teacher can see these subtle differences, and I could detect the stress in Paul Newman's legs and back before we began the movements. The relearning takes place in a subtle way, the resulting change is often subtle, but the relief can be sheer joy.

There is no need for the Alexander teacher to touch the area where strain is manifesting itself in order to assist that area. Seeing the tension in back muscles and leg muscles, the Alexander teacher works in the usual way, directing the person to go from sitting to standing and again to sitting, while lightly guiding the head and neck.

The body responds to the mental directions—at the touch of the teacher's hands. The teacher sees and feels the response immediately. Tension in the legs, for example, is transmitted throughout the body and the release can be activated in the head-neck area, which is, according to Alexander, the area of "primary control."

Normalizing head, neck and upper back dissolves tension in the lower back, arms and legs. The teacher may add additional touching assistance at the shoulders, upper back, lower back or legs.

Some years ago I was asked to teach the Alexander Technique to a group of young actors at the Mark Taper Forum in Los Angeles, as part of their training program. Surprisingly, a number of these young people had aches and pains, in their neck, shoulders, upper back, or lower back; the majority of them had poor posture and little ease in the way they moved, despite the fact that they had all had quite extensive movement and dance training.

After three or four lessons, all of them had improved their posture, and were doing much better in all other areas of their training program, voice training, dance, gymnastics, etc. They were very excited about the new ease and ability they had acquired through lengthening and lightening their bodies the Alexander way.

Two of the young men, after the first two lessons, told me that they had been suffering from back pains which had disappeared after each Alexander lesson, and had reappeared after their performance in

Camino Real where they had to participate in a strange dance on stage every evening, and they would walk offstage holding their backs in pain. I then asked them to dance for me in their next lesson. I saw that they never gave a thought to their Alexander directions. I told them to apply their Alexander directions while dancing, no matter how strange the dance. After that, no more backaches!

Actors are people who, in effect, take off their private masks and put on others, according to the role they play. The act of taking off a personal mask is part of the mind-body work that the Alexander Technique provides. You get rid of "armoring" and body language that restricts behavior and holds, often for a lifetime, the sad story of personal hardship, responsibility, hostility, and stress. Alexander methods are excitingly effective with actors, and actors are singularly successful with Alexander training. Actors hold up the mirror for us to show what we can do for ourselves. "All the world's a stage, and all the men and women merely players."

▶ Experiencing for Yourself

You are now going to participate in the joy of becoming more alive through the mind-body approach. A lightness of the body can come through doing simple movements. Then, because you are freed of the equivalent of leg chains, back packs and body restrictors, your joy expands into all body movements, and proliferates to the mind and spirit.

By experiencing this joy, you may better understand how the simple use of the mind in instructing the body can lead to such farfetched benefits as the end of colitis, or pain from arthritis or any number of other conditions.

First, though, I would like you to repeat the chair experience of Chapter I with one slight change (pages 12 to 13). As you sit in the chair and move to a standing position, then again to a sitting position, instead of thinking of the head moving forward and up as a complete concept, think of the head moving forward and up in small steps, one tiny step at a time.

These would not be spasmodic jerks of the head. These would be a continuous movement, a series of small motions upwards. This refinement of your thoughts leads to a refinement of the movement.

I'll pause now to permit you to review the instructions in Chapter I and then to do the standing/sitting movements once or twice with your mind directing your body. Remember, this experience is the gateway to limitless joy. The thoughts are of the neck being free, the head moving forward and up in small steps, and the back elongating upwards.

Perhaps you have found through more familiarity that this time your body lifted from the chair and returned to the chair with greater ease and less effort and "it made more sense."

This feeling will increase as you progress through the movements I will share with you as we travel together through these pages. I will try to project my "self" and my "touch" through these pages as warmly as possible to compensate for this distance between us, so that your periods of "doing" will bear fruit.

A major difference between self-experience and experience with a teacher is that the thoughts of "head forward and up" become automatic much faster with the teacher. By yourself, you will find you need to think these thoughts repeatedly for an extended period of time. After a series of Alexander lessons with a teacher, the body reacts automatically without your having to consciously remember the thoughts. The change comes faster. The body restores itself to its original state, before the warping had started.

▶ A Special Movement That Helps the Back

Here is a very gentle exercise that utilizes the basic approach of the Alexander Technique but is not part of the program. It is excellent for backache, tension between the shoulder blades, and stiffness in the neck.

The basic approach of the Alexander Technique is, as you now know, *ease*. It is nontrying. It is gentleness, not effort. I would like you to bring the same ease and effortlessness to this movement.

This gentle movement is helpful in releasing tension and keeping the back limber. Of itself, the exercise cannot totally re-educate you, but it can bring about, as will other movements I will show you, a great deal of pleasurable relief, as well as more suppleness in the back.

When I give these exercises, I like to be quite specific and clear.

This means many words, more words than you can remember by merely reading through and putting the book down. You could keep the book by you during the movement and pause to read the next step, or you could tape your voice reading the exercise to yourself slowly, or somebody else can help you by reading aloud from the book. I recommend taping. I also recommend doing the exercise with one or several friends.

In a moment I am going to ask you to lie on the floor on your back. Before you do, think about how you are going to move from where you are now sitting to reach a prone position on the floor. If the floor is not carpeted will you be getting a blanket or some other cushioning? (Floor padding of some kind is recommended for comfort.) Which route will you take? Will you use your hands on the chair to help you to a standing position? How will you descend to the floor? Figure out the easiest way for you. You are not going to fall to the floor like a lead weight, but what exactly are you going to do to get there? First, *visualize* yourself doing it, slowly and gently. See yourself taking your time, even *wasting your time*.

Now that you have visualized the movement, proceed with it, slowly coming to a lying position on the floor on your back.

Are you comfortable? Here is how you can be even more comfortable: slowly bend one leg so that the knee is bent and the sole of the foot is on the floor. Do the same with the other leg so that both knees are now up and both feet are on the floor.

Slowly step to the side with one foot and then with the other, so that the distance between your feet is approximately the same as the width of your shoulders. Raise your head to see how far apart your feet and knees really are. Frequently, students will place their feet only about 12 inches apart, but the shoulders are wider than that. That is because our body does not always do what we think it is doing. Put your head back on the floor. This is an excellent resting position for the back, lying with the knees bent, legs and feet apart.

Now become aware of the area of your back which you know as the waist. Gently lift that part of your back off the floor slightly and lower it again. Imagine that somebody has taken ahold of the front of your belt and is pulling you up a little bit. Use your imagination as you "permit" that part of your back to rise gently.

Your hands lie palms down, arms alongside your body. They play no part in this, nor do your buttocks. The buttocks do not rise, nor does the tail bone. Only the back of your waist responds to the imaginary tug in your belt and rises slightly off the floor. Then imagine that the tugger permits your waist to settle back on the floor.

The lift is only about one inch. Do *not* hold this position. It involves no effort, and the release involves no effort. You breathe normally. Your back muscles are doing the work, but because of your mental image, this work is done effortlessly. The lesson of effortless movement is being "learned" by these muscles.

Repeat this only five or six times. Let it become a gentle rocking motion of your pelvis. Do you feel the movement going all the way up to your head? Can you feel your spine moving gently up and down

PELVIC ROCK

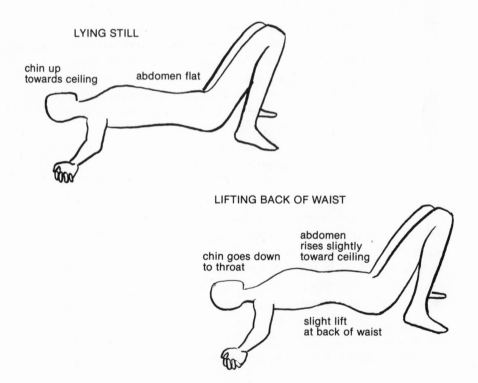

LYING STILL

chin up towards ceiling

abdomen flat

LIFTING BACK OF WAIST

abdomen rises slightly toward ceiling

chin goes down to throat

slight lift at back of waist

Note: This exercise-movement is to be done with arms alongside your body.
Doing it with arms spread out is a variation of the basic movement.

on the floor? Can you sense that your head and chin are also gently rocking? Lie still.

Slowly lower one leg to the floor and then the other, keeping them spread apart. I call this little movement a "miracle" movement for the lower back. It can eliminate tiredness, tension and aching in the lower back, as well as bringing more limberness to the muscles.

I would like next to demonstrate a subtle feeling to you. It is a good practice to become aware of subtle body feelings. Feet apart is more relaxed, in most positions and movements, than feet together, and I would like you to find this out for yourself. In a moment I will ask you to bring your feet together. First be aware of your thighs.

Bring your attention to your inner thigh muscles. Now bring your legs together, moving them one at a time or both together (moving them one at a time is easier), noticing how the inner thigh muscles work to do the movement. Notice, too, how they continue to work to hold the legs together.

Gently spread the legs again. Once your legs are apart, the muscles are able to go "off duty." Notice how relaxed they are.

This is a restful position in between doing exercises where your knees are bent. Rest your legs while on your back, arms at your sides, legs apart. You will want to enjoy this for a few minutes of restful interlude whenever you do movements with the knees bent.

At other times, it is more restful to lie on your back with knees bent, and legs and feet apart.

▶ Getting in Touch With Your Back Muscles

You may be doing some weird things with your back which you are not aware of. Becoming aware of these mannerisms would be of more than passing importance. Becoming aware of certain muscles, as you became aware of your inner thigh muscles just now, is the beginning of a new relationship between you and that part of your body.

It is like getting in touch with another person, especially an old friend. There is the establishing of communication. You begin to make changes in your movements because of this communication.

Let us do some of this establishing of communications with your back muscles while you are still lying on the floor.

You are prone, your legs lying on the floor, feet apart, arms alongside your body. Remember which knee you first lifted before? Slowly, raise the other one first this time, then slowly bring the second leg up, feet apart, soles flat on the floor, and fairly close to your buttocks. The legs and feet are apart, approximately the same width as the width of your shoulders. How did it feel to bring up the other leg first?

Bring your attention to your lower back. Notice how it is placed on the floor? And are you still breathing normally? Keeping your awareness on the muscles of your lower back, slowly lower your legs one at a time to the floor, noticing how your lower back muscles participate in the motion. Now that your legs are flat on the floor, notice how your back is placed on the floor compared to the way it was with knees up.

Still being aware of your lower back muscles and breathing normally, return your knees one at a time to the vertical position. Again, compare the way the back is lying on the floor. I think you will agree that the lower back muscles are more relaxed when the knees are up.

A release of the lower back muscles takes place when the knees are up. Utilize this "secret" between you and your lower back muscles whenever you wish to rest your back. Rest with your knees up and with your legs and feet apart.

Another "secret" you can share with your lower back muscles is that bending one knee at a time is far easier on these muscles than raising both legs simultaneously. Try it both ways and compare. Slowly lower your legs. Now raise both knees together. Slowly lower your legs. Now raise one knee at a time. I am sure you will agree one at a time was much easier, both on the back and on the legs. What is easier for the back is easier for the legs.

These are two simple insights into the functioning of your back muscles. You gain two direct benefits.

First, when you lie down to rest, *knees up is a more restful position for the back*, and secondly, when you raise them up, do so *one at a time*.

There is more benefit involved. You are in touch with your back. Being in touch with your back may reduce the need for your back to "scream" at you. As you become more and more in touch with your back, the chances of backache, back strain, and back complaints are decreased.

A few tips for greater effectiveness of the movements:

1. Move gently and slowly.
2. Do not rush.
3. Maintain your awareness, centered on wherever the directions specify.
4. Leave your eyes open.
5. Breathe at a normal, effortless rate. Optional: mouth open while exhaling.
6. Be effortless—no trying or exerting.

When doing movements as gently and easily as this, you may wonder whether you will get any benefit. Trust me. In our society, this is a new way to learn, and you are not used to it. When you become used to it, you may never want to use the old way again. The gentle, slight, slow movements can bring a pleasure and a suppleness to your body beyond anything you have know before—and then you will be "hooked." By being open and willing to experiment with a different approach, you will find that doing less gives you more— more improvement, more awareness, more insight, more understanding, more pleasure, more of what you have dreamed of.

A word about the breathing. Muscles relax more on the exhalation. They yield when you breathe out. It is best to inhale with mouth closed, or almost closed, using the nostrils and taking advantage of the tiny hairs there that filter out dust and foreign particles. Opening the mouth for the exhalation allows a fuller exhalation and a greater release in the muscles.

A final birds-eye view of this back exercise may be meaningful at this point. Notice how the lifting and lowering of the waist moved the pelvis. You might call this exercise "the Pelvic Rock." This *gentle* pelvic rock is the key to the physical effect. *Its gentleness is important.* If done forcefully, its benefits fly out the window and strain can be added instead of tension dissolved. *Gentleness makes it pleasurable, and good feelings are therapeutic.*

It can be repeated a few times, but don't overdo it. Stop while it still feels good. Then, while resting with your legs lowered to the floor, count your breaths, while breathing normally, remaining for three breaths or longer before going on to the next movement or your next activity. This is borrowed from an ancient Chinese practice: *Wait for three breaths before going to the next thing.*

While resting, take mental note of your back. Be aware of your *lower* back. How does it feel? How is it resting on the floor? Is there any difference in the way it feels *after* having done the movements? Continue up your back, feeling the sensation on the floor of each part of it. As you travel up your back, ask yourself a question: Is any part of my back lying differently on the floor from before? How do my shoulder blades lie? The back of my head? My arms? My lower back? My legs?

These changes are often subtle. As you repeat these and other movements we will be doing together, you will find these changes becoming more apparent.

This is no idle "chatter." It is meaningful "communication" between you and your back. It is *you* in touch with *your back*.

▶ Increasing Body Awareness

If you were to put the book down for a moment, close your eyes, relax and concentrate your awareness on your scalp, you would feel a slight tingling, or a warmth.

You could feel the same tingling or warmth in your hand or any part of the body to which you turn your awareness. This is going on all the time, but we are not conscious of it because our awareness is devoted to other matters. But it is there. And we can be sure that it is there merely by desiring to feel it.

You have now become aware of your back in ways that are different from the past. Previously, the back had to shout at you or pinch you in order for you to acknowledge it. Awareness of your back is beginning to move to a more sensitive level. The payoff is that you will be hearing what your back whispers to you, and this can prevent ineffable harm to your back and your entire body. The most important thing for a body that works well is to have a back that functions properly. This includes the relationship of the head to the back. The head needs to sit freely on the top of the spine. It needs to be poised lightly and in balance.

This body consciousness is among the first benefits that accrue to the Alexander student. Little tensions "speak up" which may not have been noticed before, and you let go of them. You become aware of the way you are moving and slight changes accompany that awareness in the direction of naturalness.

The Alexander Technique is a sophisticated form of rehabilitation, a relearning. A body that has been misused for 40 or 50 years *can* return to its natural movements and positions of ease and efficiency after only relatively few half-hour lessons. Your body alignment changes. Your head moves up from the top of your spine. Your spine lengthens as it relinquishes abnormal curves. Your supportive musculature becomes more dynamically balanced.

This is the essence of yourself. The essence of you lies between the top of your head and the soles of your feet.

▶ Awareness Through Movement

Just as there are many ways to teach the body misuse, there are many approaches to good use. Body awareness is being taught in a number of ways. One other to which I am devoted is the Feldenkrais method of body movement. It is called "Awareness Through Movement."

Dr. Moshe Feldenkrais, now in his mid-seventies, first developed his system in Israel more than 40 years ago. A former physicist and judo expert, he combined the body and the mind in his method, producing a marvelously effective psychophysical approach that can go alongside the Alexander Technique.

The beauty of Feldenkrais' Awareness Through Movement is that, through an ingenious variety of rolling, turning, bending and rocking exercises, as well as some very subtle exercises, combined with deep breathing, the body is reeducated. Fixed body habits are released and the body becomes incredibly supple. Through the resulting increase of energy flow, better balance and posture, and the ease of movement, a new level of fulfillment of one's potential is reached.

I first came across the Feldenkrais Method in Israel in the late 1950's. I was temporarily living in Israel and I enrolled in a Feldenkrais class. I was the youngest (and stiffest) of the students. (This was *before* I had had any Alexander lessons.) The Director of the Ministry of Education, a stocky man in his fifties who had never been particularly athletic, was one of the students in my class, and even he did better in the beginning than I did. However, I did feel very much better after each class, and as time went by I became extremely supple in the movements and noticed that I had better balance.

Feldenkrais, who had taken Alexander lessons may years ago with Alexander himself, places the emphasis on improving the back muscles. He knows that the great intrinsic strength of the back must be tapped for total efficient body usage. The exercise-movements I am giving you in this book are using the Feldenkrais approach, which goes hand-in-hand with the Alexander philosophy.

Today, with the combination of Alexander and Feldenkrais, I enjoy my body in a way that I never did before. You can experience the joy in just a few minutes a day while reading this book and applying the movements I am sharing with you.

Chapter 3

How The Alexander Technique Started

How Alexander Made His Discovery

F. MATTHIAS ALEXANDER was born in Australia, in 1869. By his early twenties, he had become a professional reciter, specializing in Shakespeare. Then trouble started. He was having difficulty with his voice while reciting on stage. His voice became increasingly hoarse and his breathing became impeded. His audiences could hear him sucking in air as he paused for breath. Alexander's throat specialist diagnosed inflammation of the vocal chords, and irritation of the mucous linings of his nose and throat. He prescribed the usual treatment of sprays and inhalants, which brought relief. However, he could not find a cause for the problem, therefore could not prescribe a cure. The condition worsened. One evening, half way through his recitation his voice was almost inaudible, by the end of the recitation he had no voice left.

He went from doctor to doctor, to no avail. Not one of them saw anything wrong that could cause such hoarseness and loss of voice. With an astuteness that was part of his personality, Alexander realized that there must be something wrong that he was doing on stage, as he did not suffer from voice difficulties at any other time. Alexander resolved to discover for himself what he was doing while reciting that brought on the symptoms.

He did not approach the problem by studying medicine. That was the physician's part, and it had not led to a solution. He began by self-observation. He stood in front of a mirror and watched himself as he prepared to recite. To his surprise, he saw that he was pulling his head downwards. When he started to recite this forced him to breathe forcefully through his mouth, and he was depressing his larnyx. Later, he noticed that he did these three things also while merely talking, only it was very slight. When he was reciting, all three actions became more exaggerated. He tried dealing with these three activities one at a time, but found he could not control them either separately or together. He then tried moving his head—first backward, then forward. The movement of the head did indeed affect these other matters.

He found that the backward movement was not an improvement, but the forward movement was. However, if he moved his head forward too much, it moved down and at this point the benefits stopped. This led him to the forward and up position of the head as the ideal one for him. He was literally making headway. Then he found that when he was pulling the head back and causing the symptoms, this was causing his chest to lift and this in turn caused the back to narrow and, in the process, his stature to shorten. The head and neck were not alone in this picture, he reasoned. The whole torso was involved. He observed himself in the mirror and saw that his back was shorter and narrower. When he moved his head to a place that looked "right" to him, forward and up, the back released and became longer and broader. Thus it was that he found the best conditions to use his voice were with the head forward and up and the back lengthening and widening.

Now what he had to do was find a way to train himself to conform to this new posture while reciting. Alexander was now aware of both the problem and the solution. This was a giant step forward, but months of disappointment still faced him. Part of the problem was that the posture that looked right in the mirror and brought about the desired release, *felt* wrong. The posture that looked wrong, *felt* right. In other words, when he *felt* that he was standing up straight and his head was going up, his breathing became difficult and the mirror showed him something that obviously looked wrong—head backwards and downwards, tight neck, and a sway back that was short and narrow. When he did what looked right in the mirror, and gave him a feeling of ease he did *not* feel that he was standing up straight.

He would practice the new alignment before reciting, but then the old alignment would persist in recurring while he was reciting.

His wrong use was habitual. Each time he decided to recite he triggered a response in his body to stand the way he always had stood for reciting because it *felt* right. Whenever the time came to use his voice and he consciously tried to do the improved head-neck position, he would find himself doing the old unwanted position again. Obviously some ingredient was lacking. He decided that the ingredient was training, that he needed to practice the new head and neck movements for a much longer period. This he did. But to his dismay when he again began to recite, he failed more often than he succeeded.

Then Alexander made a key discovery. "Up to that time the stimulus of a decision to gain a certain end had always resulted in the same habitual activity," he explains in his book *The Use of the Self.* But "as long as the reasoned directions for the bringing about of new directions were consciously maintained," then the result would be different. That meant he must not consciously decide to recite. This decision always triggered the undesirable response.

It also meant he had to give himself the instructions "head forward and up," and recite *only* when the reciting began spontaneously, as a thought rather than a decision.

By eliminating the decision to "do" an activity, in his case to recite, the old habit was bypassed. It was the decision to "do" that had triggered the unwanted responses. By substituting an allowing of the activity while primarily thinking "head forward and up" directions, Alexander finally became free of the throat and vocal trouble and of the respiratory and nasal difficulties that had plagued him for so long.

Alexander later used the word "inhibition" for the process of eliminating the decision to "do." This use of the word inhibition is as described in the dictionary: "the act or an instance of formally forbidding or barring something from being done."

Alexander spent nine years meticulously observing himself and reeducating himself with the help of a three-way mirror. Alexander would say later in his career that what took him nine years would take three months with a trained Alexander teacher.

While improving himself, he became aware that other people did similar things with their bodies. It became clear to him that whatever the poor habits, or poor posture, it always involved a rigidity in the head-neck area. As he worked on himself and on others, he found that unlocking the head-neck tension was the key to full freedom and good use of the body. He eventually called this the Primary Control.

In 1894 Alexander was officially teaching his work to others, and in 1905 he moved to England at the request of several important personalities who had heard of the unique benefits of his work. He died in 1955 in England at the age of 86.

➡ Alexander The Person

I never knew Alexander, yet I have a vivid picture of the man. This has been derived from other people's descriptions who did know him and from photographs in such books as Lulie Westfeldt's *F. Matthias Alexander, The Man And His Work* and *Body Awareness in Action—A Study of the Alexander Technique* by Frank Pierce Jones. I also saw a five-minute motion picture of Alexander shot when he was about 83 years old. Even at that age, two years after suffering a stroke from which he had fully recovered, Alexander looked alert, alive and dapper. He was teaching fulltime. He stood erect. His face was mobile and expressive. He had a distinguished, man-of-importance look, despite his short stature. He did not look up at those taller than him by turning his face up and pulling his head backwards and downwards. Instead, he raised his eyelids, as is clear in the photos in the above-mentioned books.*

All through his career Alexander was a wit and his teaching was punctuated with jokes, amusing anecdotes and quick repartee. He loved horse racing, a favorite Australian sport.

Alexander always retained an interest in acting. Part of Alexander's training of other teachers involved the students going to shows and films and the following day sharing critique, not only on

*See Bibliography

the plots and the acting, but also on the way the head-neck-back, or primary control, was functioning in the actors.

➡ His First Training Course

Alexander's teaching started long before his training of others. In fact, he resisted for decades the idea that he could train others to do what had taken so many years of his life to discover. Lulie Westfeldt described the first training in her book *F. Matthias Alexander, the Man and His Work.* Lulie was an American who had taken lessons from Alexander to help overcome the ravages of polio. Two years later, she heard that the first training course would be given in London. That was in 1931, when Alexander was 62. It took a lot of courage to invest two thousand five hundred dollars and three years in a profession that was new and virtually unknown. She later became the first Alexander teacher in New York.

Seven people that started that first training course were joined later by five more. Of the 12, three were from the United States, seven from England and two from Scotland. The ages ranged from 16 to 35. The trainees had to stand for most of the daily two-hour morning sessions as there were few chairs. But they were eager to observe as Alexander worked with each one in turn. After the completion of the first training course, Alexander continued to train. Now Alexander had teachers as assistants, and eventually left most of the training in their capable hands. He always, however, visited the training class daily and worked briefly with each trainee.

Many of the Alexander-trained teachers of those first training classes are still teaching and are today the prime source of information about the man.

Before he died in 1955, Alexander had trained others for about twenty years. Since there was only one training class every three years with an average of 10 to 15 trainees there were quite likely only about 100 who could say they were trained personally by Alexander. This left a rather small group of disciples to carry on his work.

I have personally known six of them: Patrick Macdonald, Walter and Dyllis Carrington, Marjorie Barstow, Rome Roberts, and Douglas Price-Williams who is no longer a practicing teacher having turned to psychology, but remains an ardent enthusiast of the Technique.

Edward Maisel's book *Resurrection of the Body* has a section on Alexander's sayings. "If this feels wrong to you, smile and be pleased. If you are not, leave. And don't come back until you are." This is one of the many unusual things Alexander would say while teaching. His approach to learning was revolutionary—yet very familiar to those who have studied Zen and other Eastern philosophies.

The remarkable similarity between Zen training and Alexander training is clearly revealed by reading *Zen in the Art of Archery* by Eugen Herrigel. Alexander had had no knowledge of Eastern philosophies when he developed his work. This remarkable man developed a method of learning and growth during the repressive Victorian era that is akin to philosophies of the East that are thousands of years old. Alexander was the first Westerner in recent centuries to become aware of the mind-body relationship and his work is the forerunner of the mind-body philosophies and methods that abound today in the West.

Judith Liebowitz, Director of the Alexander Center in New York, took lessons from Alexander in London two years before his death. "His hands were soft as butter," she says. Another described his touch as "soft as lambswool."

One gets a sense of a combination of firmness in the man as well as softness, of determination, of domination one time, submission the next, of impatience and patience.

Even his hands vacillated from the softness of "butter" and of "lambswool" to a firmness that the situation seemed to call for.

Alexander was quoted by the London *News Chronicle* in an interview featured in 1953 as saying, "I would like to get my hands on the statesmen of the world." Had he gotten his hands on Adolph Hitler twenty years earlier, who knows how history may have been altered.

A changed body produces a changed mind.

"I am not a healer," he said in that interview, "I am an 'educationist.' "

➡️ His Impact on His Contemporaries

Bernard Shaw wrote of Alexander, after having had lessons with him: "He established not only the beginnings of a far-reaching science of the involuntary movements . . . but a technique of correction and self control which forms a substantial addition to our very slender resources in personal education."

Sir Stafford Cripps, for several years Chancellor of the Exchequer (which is the British equivalent of our Secretary of the Treasury), was a student of Alexander's who later set up a Foundation for the Alexander Technique in England. He was quoted as saying: "Instead of feeling one's body to be an aggregation of ill-fitting parts . . . the body becomes a coordinated whole."

In his Introduction to Alexander's book, *The Use of the Self*, Professor John Dewey wrote, "If there can be developed a technique which will enable individuals really to secure the right use of themselves, then the factor on which depends the final use of all other forms of energy will be brought under control. Mr. Alexander has evolved this technique."

Dewey saw the subtlety of Alexander's work as world-shaking. Control the energy in your body efficiently and you control the world's energy more efficiently, too, Dewey was implying.

Man's consciousness is the key to his "world." Educators and sociologists are recognizing more than ever the importance of education over legislation in moving toward higher levels of life quality.

Alexander was leery of the scientists of his day. He was a loner in his field. He saw scientists as being too analytical, dividing man and matter into its components and in the process losing sight of the whole man.

Yet there were scientists who had only words of praise for Alexander. Among them were Sir Charles Sherrington, a great British neurophysiologist and Nobel Prize winner, and the renowned American biologist, Charles E. Coghill, and more recently, Professor Nikolaas Tinbergen, Nobel Laureate.

Said Professor Coghill, "Mr. Alexander's method lays hold of the individual as a whole, as a self-vitalizing agent. He reconditions and reeducates the reflex mechanisms and brings their habits into normal relation with the functions of organisms as a whole. I regard his methods as thoroughly scientific and educationally sound."

In the field of the intellectuals of his day he found his greatest authoritative supporters. Aldous Huxley was among them. Said Huxley: "Mind and body are organically one; and it is therefore inherently likely that, if we can learn the art of conscious inhibition on the physical level, it will help us acquire and practice the same art on the emotional and intellectual levels. A good physical education will be one which I have called preventive ethics, forestalling many kinds of trouble by never giving them the opportunity to arise.

"So far as I am aware, the only system of physical education which fulfills all these conditions is the system developed by F.M. Alexander."

Huxley included descriptions of the Technique in every book he wrote since his lessons with Alexander.

Educator John Dewey contributed to introducing the philosophy of the Alexander Technique to America, after he had taken lessons with Alexander during his stay in the United States.

"Education is the only sure method which mankind possesses for directing his own course. But we have been involved in a vicious circle. Without knowledge of what constitutes a truly normal and healthy psycho-physical life, our professed education is likely to be miseducation. The technique of Mr. Alexander gives to the educator a standard of psychophysical health, in which what we call morality is included."

On February 26th, 1953, the *News Chronicle* of London printed an article, in a section entitled People Worth Meeting, called "He Teaches The Way Back To Health," by Ronald Searle and Kaye Webb. The article was a combination of a description of F.M. Alexander and an interview with him. The article describes how, at the beginning of the century, Sir Henry Irving, the great British actor of that time, would call on Mr. Alexander to help him. It refers to George Bernard Shaw's recuperation to health from angina at the hands of Alexander, and how the only person sitting up straight in the House of Lords after an all-night session was another pupil of Alexander's, Lord Lytton. The article goes on to describe how Alexander, in the process of trying to cure his voice problem, discovered "that my *feeling*, the only guide I had to depend on for the direction of my use, was untrustworthy . . ." To quote a section from the article: "His final discovery of what he has called 'the means whereby' meant a complete reeducation in the use of the human body. It achieved what had before seemed impossible, 'it bridged the gap between the subconscious and the unconscious.' "

Closer to our day, Edward Maisel, Director of the American Physical Fitness Research Institute, wrote: "We learn from this technique a definite way of adapting ourselves to our environment, no matter what we may be doing. We apply ourselves, henceforth, by means of a new kinesthetic experience involving head, neck and trunk. We proceed with a fresh overall sensation of lightness and ease in the handling of our bodies."

▶ An Alexander "Experience"

Perhaps, through the following gentle head movement, with my guidance I can help you have a taste of this "kinesthetic experience . . . of lightness and ease."

Stand as comfortably as you can, with your feet comfortably apart, your arms hanging comfortably at your sides, and look ahead easily. Turn your head to the right, and turn your head to the left and come back to the middle. Do this again, turning your head right and left, and see whether you are moving your shoulders and whether your upper torso is turning as you turn your head. If you are, I would like you to do it now *without* moving your shoulders or torso. Move only your head right and left. Move it gently, without straining. Go only as far as is comfortable. Mark an imaginary spot on the wall on your right as your landmark, to show how far you turned your head to the right, and do the same on your left. Let your head come to the middle.

Think of the instances in your daily life when you turn your head. It is when you want to look at something. You may turn your head when you hear a sound, but you are turning *to see* where that sound came from or what the sound is about. It is only natural that your eyes lead the movement, as it is the eyes that you see with.

I would like you now to gently turn your eyes to the right and allow your head to follow, and perhaps you have gone past your landmark on the wall. If you have, mark a new imaginary spot on the wall. Now gently turn your eyes to the left and let your head follow your eyes, and see how far you go to the left. Perhaps here, too, you have gone past your landmark and can mark a new one on the wall. Turn your head right and left a few times with your eyes leading. Enjoy the movement, let it be light and pleasurable. Is there a nicer quality in the movement? We are interested in improving quality, and with that often comes an increase in quantity.

When we use ourselves in a way that is more functional, and with greater awareness, which is the same as better use, we can improve our functions; when we move in a mindless way, we are much more limited. Turning your head in a mindless compulsive way not only limits the movement, but it is done with more strain in the neck muscles, and the neck muscles are connected to the shoulder muscles, and the shoulder muscles are connected to your back muscles, and the strain travels all the way down your body to your feet.

Now let us do this movement with Alexander directions. Again, I would like your eyes to lead. Before you start moving your eyes and head, say lightly to yourself, "head forward and up, back lengthening," and continue having those thoughts in mind as you gently let your head and eyes turn to the right. Perhaps you actually felt yourself lengthen, become taller and lighter; and perhaps you have gone past both of your landmarks with ease. If you have, then you can mark a new imaginary spot on the wall.

Again, gently give yourself the thought of your head going forward and up and your back lengthening, and repeating the thoughts lightly let your eyes and head turn to the left, and see how far you go to the left, and see whether you feel the kinesthetic lightness that you can have with Alexander directions. Have you gone past your second landmark? If you have, mark a new one on the wall. Turn right and left a few times this way, lightly and gently (*not rushing through it*), and directing *before, during, and after* each part of the movement. Be aware of any differences in the way you feel. Now let your head stay in the middle. Do it again in the same way that you just did with your Alexander directions, turning only to the right. This time go only as far as your first landmark. Give your Alexander directions again easily, and gently turn your eyes and head further to the right, and see whether you go to your third landmark, and perhaps you may even be going beyond it. What I would like you to notice is how much increase you got in the movement between the first time you did it and this last time. Do the same thing to the left, and before you start moving give your Alexander directions, head forward and up, back lengthening, and have those thoughts in mind as you gently let your eyes and head turn to the left, and stop at your first landmark. Give your Alexander directions again easily, eyes and head turn further to the left, and see how far you go now. See how much increase you have on the left. And come back to the front.

Now gently move into walking. See whether the greater ease, lightness and lengthening has carried over into your walking. Does your head feel as if it is poised lightly on top of your spine? Does your back feel longer and lighter? Are your legs freer?

You may want to repeat this Alexander "experience" while sitting on a chair, and when you finish come up to standing and walk around and see if you have a taste of that "fresh overall sensation of lightness and ease."

➡ The First Minutes of an Alexander Lesson

A man in his fifties was not sure whether he wanted to take Alexander lessons. "I have heard nice things about it, but can you give me a few minutes of your time and perhaps a brief demonstration?"

I agreed. The following is a taping of those few minutes.

"Looking at you, I see you don't have any serious problems of misalignment. There are some relatively slight things I see. Your left leg has more tension in it than the right leg. I notice a slight sway back, very slight. Your shoulders are fairly level. You seem to have your greatest tension in your legs and some in your lower back. I would say that nothing bothers you, no aches or pains. You don't look to me as if you have any.

"What I usually do first is have people look at themselves in the mirror. Most people who come for lessons have distortions in their alignment. One shoulder higher than the other, one hip higher, a sway back, or hunched shoulders, and various other things. After the lesson they can look again to make a comparison. In your case, you won't see great changes in the mirror, because your misalignment is slight.

"However, I do see some tensions and they are primarily in the legs; you tend to lock your knees. And you push your calves backwards (you hyperextend your legs). It's what is commonly called 'saber legs.' They curve backwards. And the arches of your feet fall inwards. If you'll look at your feet, I think you'll see that. I'm not looking so much at the direction in which your feet are pointed but at how the arches are falling inwards and downwards, instead of upwards.

"My feet used to be very much like that. I don't have fantastically high arches now, and I never will have, but I do have a fairly decent arch as the result of the Alexander work.

"It's not only your feet that have tension. Your legs also have tension. That is a result of pulling the torso downwards instead of letting it go upwards against gravity. You are pulling yourself down with gravity.

"The end result of all that weight bearing down is stress on your legs and feet. In the Alexander work, we don't try to correct feet or legs. We teach people how to direct the muscles and spine of the whole torso to go upwards, which is what they are supposed to be doing naturally. It's through misuse that we pull ourselves downwards. Some people *strain* to push upwards.

"When we use ourselves well, the long muscles in the torso, and the neck muscles, do their job well. They hold us up against gravity easily and effortlessly. When they're not . . . we pull ourselves down with gravity. The majority of people start showing it in the shoulders, then in the back by slumping, arching the back, and causing tension in the legs and feet. In your case, it doesn't seem to be affecting your torso as much as your legs and feet.

"However, you do have a slight sway back. Right in here. Very gently put your tail back and slightly arch your back so that you feel the exaggeration of your sway back. Now stand as you normally do. Now I don't want you to change the way you usually stand. Let your hands hang down normally.

"Now I would like you to sit on the table facing the window. Bring your legs up on the table. Your job is to do nothing except to think certain thoughts. Allow *me* to move *you*. I don't want you to get involved with the movements, only give the thoughts 'Let the neck be free, to let the head go forward and up, to let the back lengthen and widen.'

"Good. I felt the effect of your thoughts. I don't like to use the term relax, but I also don't want you to think of working at this. I don't want you to work; instead, let yourself be in a neutral state.

"I realize that for most people sitting in this position is difficult at first. I won't keep you here for long. After some Alexander lessons you will be able to sit like this quite comfortably. My aim is not to keep you here very long, just enough to give you some instructions.

"I want you to think of your head floating up to the ceiling, as if your head were a balloon. And without staring; I don't want you to get into a fixed stare. Think of the top of your head floating up like a balloon and touching the ceiling *a little ahead*.

"The head going up, *forward* and *up*. Think of your spine lengthening upwards. The spine goes up, the head goes forward and up, and it's going up in a slight curve. Just give that thought again and again, lightly and easily. And you can say to yourself the words that are defining those thoughts. 'Let the neck be free to let the head go forward and up to let the back lengthen and widen.'

"Now forget about the ceiling and the lengthening upwards and let me move you to a lying position on the table. You now need to tell your hip joints to release. Yes, it happened. Think of your spine lengthening *out* along the table. *Not* down, *out*! Only *think* these things, please don't try to do them.

"You're a little afraid to give me your full weight. When I am taking you down to lie on the table, you can give me your full weight.

"Good! You see, when you're thinking about length, you are not heavy at all.

"I am going to do everything for you. I will ask you only to give these lengthening directions to the spine, the back, and the whole torso. They are elastic, getting longer and longer, following the head as it goes out. And I would like you to give your thoughts lightly and easily. This is *not* a heavy concentration.

"Lightly and easily, and without caring whether it works or not, or whether you're doing the right thing. Simply give your thoughts.

Now I'm going to move your legs to make you more comfortable. Let *me* do it. You don't need to care about your legs or your arms. Your job is to care about your head going out towards the wall behind you and your back lengthening and widening.

"I will remind you again and again, and I will say the words over and over. You can say the words silently to yourself. Let the neck be free, to let the head go forward and out, to let the back lengthen and widen. Don't get into a fixed stare; blink your eyes normally and move your eyes a little to look at different spots on the ceiling, and breathe as usual.

"Your head is going forward and out, your back lengthening and widening. Think of your length. I don't want you to think of the leg that I'm moving for you. I will take care of the leg, and you take care of directing your head and back. Good. Now think of your length again, head going out, back lengthening and widening. Good. I felt your direction and your leg moved easily.

"Let the neck be free to let the head go forward and out. I sense that you are now getting used to doing nothing, allowing your head to go out, leading the lengthening of your back."

In five minutes this man was responding in ways that were visually evident to me and evident in a feeling way to him. I followed the "table work" with "chair work," applying the Alexander directions to sitting and standing and walking: "Neck free, head forward and *up*, back lengthening and widening."

He made an appointment for a second lesson.

That is the beginning of the Alexander Technique.

Chapter 4

Conditions
That Respond
to the Technique

PROFESSOR NIKOLAAS TINBERGEN received the Nobel Prize for Physiology or Medicine, together with K. Lorenz and K. von Frisch, on December 12, 1973. His lecture, on the occasion of accepting the prize, was entitled "Ethology and Stress Diseases,"* and was partially devoted to the Alexander Technique. After explaining how he and two other members of his family went to three different Alexander teachers for lessons he continued: " . . . the evidence given and documented by Alexander . . . of beneficial effects on a variety of vital functions no longer sounds so astonishing to us. Their long list includes . . . rheumatism . . . various forms of arthritis, then respiratory troubles, and even potentially lethal asthma; following in their wake, circulation defects, which may lead to high blood pressure and also to some dangerous heart conditions; gastrointestinal disorders of many types; various gynecological conditions; sexual failures; migraines and depressive states that often lead to suicide; in short, a very wide spectrum of diseases, both somatic and mental, that are not caused by identifiable parasites."

Among the conditions that respond well to the Technique is back problems. Edward Maisel, director of the American Physical Fitness Research Institute, has written:**

*Reprinted in *Science* July 5, 1974

**"Take Inches From Your Waist—Exercise Without Exercise" *Harper's Bazaar*, April 1967

"At the Institute of Rehabilitation Medicine in New York, the technique presently figures among the resources of physiotherapy available to patients. It is being used to help alleviate selected cases of low backache, pinched nerve, scoliosis, tension syndome and certain other distortions. Dr. Allen Russek, Director of Specialized Services there, explains that such means can also be used, on occasion, as a substitute for such mechanical devices as halters, corsets, neck braces or shoulder pins: that is to say, in cases where it is possible to effect a change in the patient's center of gravity through internal shifting rather than external pressure."

The Back as a Barometer of Health

Back problems are one of the most common ailments in America and certainly the one that is least helped by standard, or allopathic, medicine.

Dr. Hans Kraus is a foremost authority on backache and back pain in the United States. He is the doctor who helped the late President Kennedy with a back problem in the last two years of his life, enabling Kennedy to play golf again. A wartime injury had interfered with his normal back movement and had caused considerable pain. After treatment from Dr. Kraus, Kennedy was able to move more freely and naturally with less pain.

Dr. Kraus has claimed that muscle spasm and muscle tension, together with the whole syndrome of neck, back, and leg pains, are due basically to poor posture. Correct your posture and postural habits, he has said, and the problems will not occur. By postural habits, he explained, he meant the simple activities we perform daily, such as talking on the telephone.

How do you hold the telephone to your ear? Do you scrunch up your shoulder with the phone there? Do you reach strenuously for it, or bend down easily to pick it up? How do you bend down at a sink to wash your hands or to pick up things? Knees together would be a poor postural habit. Knees straight makes it hard on the back muscles.

Dr. Kraus' theory is that back and related problems derive from an accumulation of these apparently minor body habits done poorly.

If there is a case for preventive medicine, the human back is its prime witness. Once a person has back problems, doctors have little to offer as a remedy.

As Alexander struggled with his own body behavior problems, he found that the body became less a system of ill-fitting parts and more of a fluid continuum, with each part related to the other through a continuous flow of impulses.

Small distortions of these impulses produce a cumulative effect of disintegration. The parts become less integrated with each other. We become a system of separate parts no longer working together. Some parts take on work not intended for them. Some do not work at all. Some develop tightness from exerting large pressures that have no purpose; others lose their tone from lack of use.

Yes, we could be put "in traction" and we might be forced back into shape. But how long would it last? The back must learn to *restore itself*. This learning can be done only through experience. Reading this book is therefore only half the story. You cannot learn to be a tea taster or a wine taster by reading a book. You need the cups of tea or the glasses of wine.

From the experience is the joy derived.

➡ A Tale of Two Backs

Milton Thomas of Los Angeles is a renowned violist with a very busy schedule. Besides his concerts and teaching he does recordings for motion picture studios. After a period of backache, he was flat on his back for three months with a ruptured disc. Any movement caused incredible pain. Several orthopedists and orthopedic surgeons agreed that the only answer was surgery. One informed him that the spinal fluid was blocked and that he would become paralyzed unless an operation was performed to correct it.

Wanting to avoid surgery, Milton called me in desperation. I went to his house and began to give him Alexander lessons while he was lying in bed. I worked even more subtly and gently with him than I usually did. After a few lessons, he was able to get out of bed. Then his wife drove him to my studio to continue the lessons. Soon he was driving himself.

After one month of lessons, three times a week, he was fully mobile again, walking and driving, and almost pain-free. He was then able to gradually resume his busy schedule of concerts, teaching, and recordings. He went back to the surgeon who had examined him a month before. The surgeon reexamined him, looked at his previous x-rays, and stated, "When you were here last I said surgery was imminent. Now I say surgery is not imminent."

After he was back in full swing with no pain whatsoever, Milton Thomas continued his Alexander lessons for several more weeks for reinforcement. It is now more than two years since his last Alexander lesson and he has not had a recurrence of the problem.

What was the bedridden Milton Thomas subjected to at the hands of his Alexander teacher to bring about his relief?

If you were there you would have seen me place my hands gently on his head and neck, which were on a pillow, and verbally give him the basic Alexander directions, as I do with every student:

"Let the neck be free, to let the head go forward and out, to let the back lengthen and widen." (When lying down, we use "head forward and *out*.")

He cooperated by thinking the directions, thinking of a released neck and of his head moving back towards the wall behind his bed. In fact, I asked him to pretend there was a large hole in the wall so that his head would move through it and out to infinity.

I asked him to imagine that his back and spine were lengthening, as if made of elastic. I explained that as the back and spine are attached to the head, they have to follow as the head goes out, and they also lengthen to infinity.

The purpose of my hands is to suggest this ever so subtly to the neck and head while at the same time detecting his response. Because of his serious condition, I did not make even the slightest movement of his head and spine with my hands. Instead, I relied purely on the message of the directions being transmitted through the light touch of my fingers. (In the case of a spinal disorder, the least movement could be disastrous.) An Alexander teacher knows how to direct and the impulses are transmitted through the hands.

That is all I did—staying at his head and saying the Alexander directions. Naturally, as an Alexander teacher, I had learned how to do this in the most effective way. Once in a while, I smoothed out his shoulders, or gently lowered and raised his legs, always with Alexander direction. You would say, if watching, that I did almost nothing. The Alexander directions, transmitted from the mind, are more powerful than physical movement.

I would bend one knee at a time, gently and slowly, while he gave these same neck, head and back thoughts to himself. This is the usual Alexander work. In his case, as his legs and back were very weak, I propped up each knee with a pillow.

Usually, there is a noticeable lengthening of the body—in fact, the books we put under the head when the student lies on the table have to be moved backwards in order to accommodate the new body length. But this was not so in the case of Milton Thomas. The changes were almost imperceptible during the first lesson. One very noticeable change was that he looked much more relaxed, much younger, and that his pale face had become rosy with improved circulation. His face was almost radiant! At the end of the lesson he said that he felt very relaxed.

After the first lessons, the back did indeed lengthen perceptibly and Milton's physical improvement began to be obvious.

Sometimes people come for Alexander lessons *after* back surgery because of continued pain.

Rose G. had had two operations on her back. In her mid-thirties, she was a petite, attractive mother of two teenage daughters and the wife of a well-to-do businessman. She worked with her husband, running the business that they owned.

She had a disc problem and scoliosis. Scoliosis is a sideways curvature of the spine. Physicians are becoming more aware of this problem in children since a large number appear to develop this problem quite early. For some reason, it is more common in girls than in boys. It usually causes no discomfort in childhood although it often makes children more awkward. It can get worse in adults as it did in the case of Rose G., and usually causes severe pain.

Her first surgery had resulted in disaster—she was in a wheelchair and could not stand or walk. There was an improvement in her condition after her second surgery. She could then move and function but she was never comfortable and felt constant pain.

Rose would rush over for Alexander lessons during her lunch hour. After her first lesson she felt a reduction in pain level. After the first three lessons, within a span of one week, she estimated that her pain was reduced by 50 percent. After about three weeks of lessons, she invited me for lunch and a swim in her pool.

There I met her husband and here is the way I was introduced. "Thanks to Judith and the Alexander Technique, I am free of pain for the first time in fifteen years." They later sent their two teenage daughters for lessons, too, as their posture was poor.

➡ A Curved Spine

Scoliosis is the name for a sideways curvature of the spine, either a C curve, or an S curve. The S curve is technically a double scoliosis, and is the more severe condition. Most people who are told they have a scoliosis have an S curve in their spine. This condition is both distorting to the body and also, in most cases, quite painful. Scoliosis can start at an early stage and is often detected in young children. The medical answers are daily exercises, a brace, or surgery. The first two often prevent further curvature in children, but not always, and only sometimes decrease the curve. On the whole, children do not enjoy repetitive exercises or a brace, and some refuse to co-operate. Surgery is a serious, risky undertaking.

The Alexander Technique, through reeducating the use of the muscles in the torso, has been very helpful in cases of scoliosis, in both adults and children. They look better, feel better, and have a better prospect for the future. And they enjoy the lessons. Several of my students have come for lessons because of the disfigurement or pain of scoliosis. With some of the children, and teenagers, before-and-after x-rays were taken, and showed a significant decrease in the curvature; in some of the adults there has been a slight decrease in the curvature. Scoliosis is considered to be progressive in most cases, constantly becoming worse. To arrest the worsening is already an improvement, and to effect a decrease in the degree of curvature is considered quite remarkable.

One 13-year-old girl was brought to me for Alexander lessons by her parents when several orthopedists insisted that her curvature was too severe to be left alone and they wanted to prescribe a brace for her. One of them agreed to wait three months and see what the Alexander Technique could do for her. The girl came two or three times each week. During the first month, her parents were telling me that not only did she look better and move more gracefully, but also her hyperactive behavior had calmed down. After three months, the orthopedist took new x-rays and announced that her curvature had decreased by 14°. Naturally, we were all very pleased with the medical confirmation of the results, but I recommended that she continue her Alexander lessons on a less intensive basis as long as she is growing, as that is the most vulnerable period with scoliosis.

I have worked with children, teenagers and adults with scoliosis, some of them after surgery that had left them in severe pain. The work has always brought about very gratifying improvement, and I know that other Alexander teachers have had similar results.

One of our Alexander teachers, in New York City, Deborah Caplan, M.A., R.P.T., has published a brochure for the medical profession, entitled: *Postural Management of Scoliosis in the Adolescent and Adult Based on the Alexander Technique*. In a section dealing with adolescent scoliosis she writes of improved use on a long term basis:

"Because instruction in the Alexander Technique teaches a child a system of body use whereby postural errors can be detected and eliminated, it will be of practical value throughout life. For those with scoliosis, correcting body use should be an ongoing process that takes into account the varying physical demands made on the adult—such as office work, pregnancy, sports, performing in the arts etc. . . ."

And with regard to scoliosis in the adult, Caplan writes:

"The problems that are found most frequently in adults with scoliosis are back pain, arthritic changes in the spine, and a tendency for the lateral curves to slowly increase. Because these problems are aggravated by faulty postural habits and unnecessary muscle tension, many adults with scoliosis have found studying the Alexander Technique beneficial."

Note: The thirteen-year-old girl reported her subjective experiences as follows: she was much more comfortable in sitting and standing, and all other activities. She no longer had to hem up her skirts on one side. She was so pleased with the improvement in her appearance after two months that she bought bikinis for her summer swimming.

▶ Pain as a Message From Your Body

How can people live with pain year after year? It is like letting the telephone ring and ring and not answering it. Pain is a "telephone" call from the body, an SOS, a cry for help.

So what do we do? We take an aspirin or some other pain killer. That is like taking the telephone off the hook.

Listen to the message of the body. It comes through loud and clear: "Misuse."

I met a woman at a dinner party. I could see that her back was very rigid and she did not walk easily. By the end of the evening, I could tell she was in pain.

"You seem to be in pain," I said to her.

"How can you tell?" she replied, surprised.

"That's the work I do."

She then told me how she had had three spinal fusions, and was in constant daily pain, from the moment she awakened in the morning. I told her of the Alexander Technique. "I'd like to show it to you and maybe help you." We went into another room.

I asked her to lie down on the floor and I placed a couple of books under her head, exactly as we do in the Alexander lessons. I worked with her in the way I have previously described.

After about fifteen minutes she stood up. She looked pleased. "I feel fine," she beamed. She called me a few days later and said that for two and one half days she had been totally free of pain. "It's the first time since my operation that I am without pain."

The reason she called was that the pain was gradually returning.

She wanted to start regular lessons. It took only a brief period of lessons to totally rid her of her back pain but there was pain in her shoulder that was more stubborn.

What was the "telephone" message of her shoulder? It took a bit of detective work to discover it. She swam regularly on doctor's orders. "What stroke do you use?" I asked. "The crawl," was her reply. That was the answer. The crawl would indeed affect the shoulder if she was putting too much effort into it.

The Alexander lessons had been relieving this pain, too, but as soon as the misuse of the shoulder was repeated while swimming, the poor shoulder got back on the "telephone" again.

I went to her house and swam with her in her pool, showing her how she misused her shoulders and how to swim with greater ease, and suggesting other strokes that she could do with less tension in the arm and shoulder. That was the end of her shoulder pain. Eventually, she was doing the crawl also, free of shoulder pain.

Sometimes pains persist. They are relieved during the lesson and directly afterwards but return again before the next lesson. When this is the case, I know the student is continuing to do something in his/her daily life that needs adjusting. Frequently it is something in their job or in a sports activity. I don't like to probe into people's life styles, but I don't like to leave these "telephone" calls of pain unanswered. Through questioning I find out which activity it is. Usually, we can find a better way to do it. Sometimes it is only the car seat causing back pain and that can be easily adjusted. With my students who drive a car, I ask them to drive me around a few blocks and I observe what they do as they drive, and offer better alternatives. This often eliminates a recurring ache or pain.

The back needs a whole "switchboard" for its use. It is one of the most prolific sources of pain. Yet, through the Alexander Technique—which means substituting proper use for misuse—99 percent of all back pains respond within a few lessons. Most achieve total relief after several lessons.

A woman was in a severe automobile accident. Previously, she had had recurrent lower back pains. In addition to these, since her accident she had severe pain in her upper back, shoulders and neck due to whiplash. With the Alexander Technique the lower back pain totally disappeared and did not return during the months I knew her, but the upper pain would come and go.

That meant I needed to do some detective work. I learned that she drove over 20 miles each way on the freeways to and from work. I watched her drive and I could see no obvious misuse. But she did say that turning her head to switch lanes at the freeway intersections hurt her neck and that she always drove during the rush hour. The mental stress of driving was obviously also causing physical strains. On the days she did not drive to work her neck did not hurt, even though prior to Alexander lessons it had hurt all the time. Since she would not stop driving during rush hour we could not avoid the neck strain, unless she avoided the freeways. She was not willing to give up either one, even though she was financially independent. In this case, the student chose to have the pain rather than make a change in life style. Most people prefer to make a change in their life when necessary.

Pinched nerves are another cause of continuing discomfort. Tingling and/or numbness are characteristics of their "message." This could be a severe condition. When the nerve is pinched in the neck, tingling or numbness would be felt in the arms. When it is felt in the legs, the pinched nerve would be in the lower back. I even had one case of a girl with numbness in her left buttock!

If the painful "telephone" call of a pinched nerve is not acted on, paralysis can eventually occur. The only accepted medical approach to a pinched nerve that I have heard of is an operation. If the operation is not successful, the patient may be crippled for life. The Alexander Technique, in my own practice, and in the practice of other teachers I know has not failed to relieve a case of pinched nerve.

Medicine treats the symptom instead of the cause. What movement or posture is bringing pressure to bear on a disc or pinching a nerve? Stop moving or holding your body in that way and you could remove the cause and the pain.

➡ An Exercise to Massage Your Back

There are many gentle movements that are helpful for the back muscles, and therefore for the whole body. However, there is no exercise or movement that should be done when a person is in severe pain from a disc problem, or is in muscle spasm. The answer in these cases is bed rest, and, if possible, Alexander lessons with a highly skilled teacher.

The movement I am going to share with you now is helpful for less severe back conditions, and is also a marvelously effective way to help prevent back problems. You can massage your own back and effect a release from tension in the back muscles, and perhaps you will also feel some other changes in yourself that you have not experienced before.

The movements I give in this book are small and gentle, and are to be done that way. If you find it hard to believe that such small, and seemingly insignificant movements are beneficial, think of it as an experiment. After all, I am sure that at one time or another in your life you have done strenuous activities, and you know what that feels like and what it does for you; now you can experiment with a different approach and see what it can do for you.

Find an easy way to come to lying on the floor on your back, with your legs stretched out along the floor and comfortably apart. Notice how your back is lying on the floor. Which parts lie with greater pressure against the floor and which parts lie with less pressure against the floor, are any part or parts of your back not touching the floor at all? Think of your right leg and notice how it lies against the floor, and now think of your left leg and see how it lies against the floor, and compare the two legs. Do they feel the same or do they feel different from each other? Think of the backs of your thighs, the backs of your knees, your calf muscles and your heels. And think of your toes too. Now think of the back of your head and see how the back of your head is lying against the floor, and exactly which part is making the greatest contact with the floor.

Gently draw up your legs one at a time, all the while breathing normally and not holding your breath. When your knees are bent, see that your legs and feet are spread comfortably apart, approximately the same distance as the width across your shoulders. Sense how your back lies on the floor in this position and compare it to the way it was when you had your legs down on the floor. Make a mental note of what your back feels like now so that you can remember it later.

Gently pick up your right foot. When you do this, you will find that your right knee is poised above your right hip joint. I want to call this the starting position and you can refer to my photograph below to see what this position is. Now I would like you to do a small, gentle movement with your right knee, moving it slightly towards your head and return to the starting position; do this gently a few times. The knee moves only about three or four inches, it is not a big movement. Please do it gently and at a comfortable pace, not rushing through it. Notice how this movement is working on your right hip joint, and perhaps you can also feel that your whole back is being moved up and down along the floor. Perhaps you even feel that your head is being moved. Can you sense your chin going down towards your throat and away again? These feelings are likely to be subtle.

Gradually make the size of your knee movement smaller and smaller and faster, so that eventually you are doing very tiny, very fast movements. When you are doing these very fast movements, see that you are not holding your breath. When you do these very small, fast little movements, I think that you will feel your spine and your back are being wobbled up and down the floor, and your head also. *You are massaging your back.* Allow yourself to wobble like jello.

After you have done this several times, very gently put your right foot down on the floor again. Notice whether you feel any difference in the way your back is lying on the floor and perhaps you feel a greater difference on one side than on the other side.

Very gently, lower your legs one at a time. See whether you feel some difference in the way your body lies on the floor with your legs down, and whether you feel a change on one side that is more pronounced than on the other side. Notice your legs. Does one leg feel different than the other? Does it feel smoother or longer than the other? Compare your two hip joints. Does one hip joint feel more open and freer than the other hip joint? Think of your two eyes. Does one eye feel more open than the other eye? Leave your eyes open while you are sensing your eyes. Breathe normally. Perhaps you feel a connection between your right eye and your right hip joint and your right leg?

Now gently draw up your knees one after the other. Roll over onto

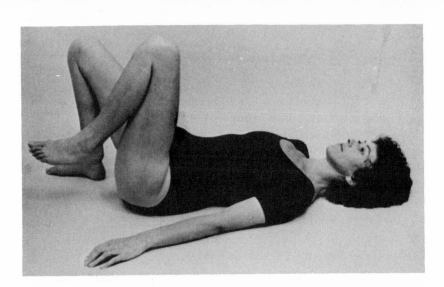

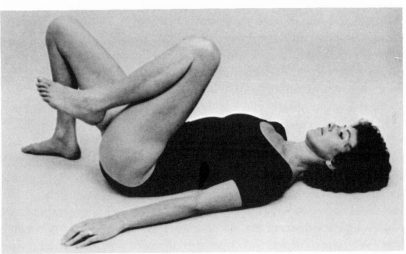

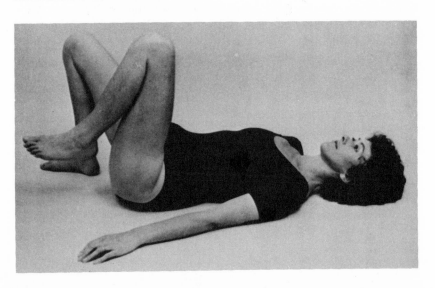

your right side, leaving your knees bent, all the way onto your hands and knees, and from there, come up to standing.

Walk around normally and notice whether one side of your body feels different to the other side. Does one side feel longer and taller? Does one hip joint feel freer? Do you feel that one side of your body seems shorter and more contracted almost as if you are a cripple on that side?

Now gently come to lying on the floor again. Draw up your knees one at a time, and spread your feet and legs apart.

This time, lift your left foot and do your gentle knee movement with your left knee. Notice how your left hip joint moves with this movement and how this gentle movement of your left knee is making your whole body move up and down the floor, including your head. Gradually allow the movement to become smaller and faster. Smaller and smaller and faster and faster, until finally you are doing very tiny fast movements which make your back wobble up and down the floor. Allow yourself to wobble like a piece of jello.

After a while, gently allow your left foot to come down to the floor again. How do you lie on the floor now?

Roll over again onto your right side, all the way onto your hands and knees, and gently come up to standing. See how you feel as you stand. Walk around and see whether your left side now feels much more like the right side, whether your whole body feels lighter. Do you feel taller? Do you feel as if you are floating or gliding rather than walking? Please don't try to change your walk. Walk normally; however, your normal walk may feel different now than what it was like before. The effects of this very gentle self-massaging of your back can give you some of the same effects as an Alexander lesson with an Alexander teacher.

➡ The Response of Psychosomatic Conditions to Alexander Lessons

Can pain be psychosomatic?

The answer can be "yes" or "no." All pain is real, whether or not it is psychosomatic. We are not asking whether the pain is imagined or not.

A definition of psychosomatic pain could be: "a pain due to a condition brought about by the person for emotional needs." For example, the only way someone can get attention from her husband or family is to be crippled by rheumatoid arthritis. Of course, such pain is psychosomatic, although the physical symptom of the ailment manifested is very real. That ailment and its pain are emotionally caused.

What about the pain of a broken rib? "Not psychosomatic" cries a unison of voices. But suppose the broken rib was incurred in an automobile accident which took place after a knockdown battle with a spouse? The accident was emotionally caused.

We can also conceivably arrive at a situation where the answer is a unanimous "no," where the pain is not psychosomatic. To do this we might have to go into the 10 percent area of inherited conditions, or a condition a person is born with, such as a clubfoot.

The person with a clubfoot or a deformed back can also misuse his or her body and could be relieved of the ensuing pain with the Alexander Technique, though, of course, not of the condition.

Emotionally caused conditions can be helped through the Alexander Technique, except for one. Even the accident-prone person can be helped by preventing the build up of tension that causes the accidents in the first place.

The person who cannot be helped is the person who demands the condition and has self-inflicted it because of the advantages it brings.

When a person psychologically causes an illness, even though not on an intentional or conscious level, that illness serves a purpose. A strong emotional need is being served by the condition. Some of those people start to get well, then they stop coming to their Alexander lessons. The incentive to get well lessens as the motivation to keep the condition for its emotional benefit is being threatened.

➡ Other Stubborn Medical Conditions that Respond

When I was practicing in New York City a lady with Parkinson's Disease, who lived in Washington, D.C., came to New York for Alexander lessons.

The disease was fairly well advanced. She shuffled and she could not speak properly. She was just short of being confined to a wheelchair.

Because she could only stay five weeks, I advised her to take lessons five times a week. She agreed, dividing the lessons among three teachers. At the end of that time the woman's speech and movement were almost normal.

A key in this dramatic improvement was her ability to direct her body with her mind. I saw this in the very first lesson. She wanted to walk toward a door or toward a chair, and as she approached her destination the shuffle became intensified.

This concern for reaching her goal, called "end gaining" by Alexander, was a contributing factor to her shuffling. By substituting different directions for this "end gaining" direction, the shuffling did *not* increase as she came closer to her goal. Eventually her shuffling was totally gone.

The instructions for her were the same as for everyone else, to direct her head forward and up and her back to lengthen as she walked. After several lessons, she did not have to give herself these directions each time. They had "taken."

We cannot say that this woman was "cured" of Parkinson's Disease, since it is a progressive disease. But the thought does linger that the progressive aspect of such a disease might be based on the reinforcement of faulty directions. Stop that chain and you may interrupt a progression and cause a quasi-permanent regression.

Another woman was referred to me by her physician. Four years before, she had suffered a head injury when a piece of falling ceiling hit her. For some time she had not been able to walk and could only crawl like a baby.

After four years of medical treatment and physical therapy, her doctors were finally able to get her back on her feet. She could stand and walk again but she lurched. If she headed across the room toward a door she would end up in another part of the room. You would have thought she was drunk. She also fell frequently, without any reason. When she stood, she had to brace her legs by spreading her legs apart and standing on the inside edges of her feet. To get out of her chair, she pressed on her knees with her hands until, after several minutes, with great effort, she made it. Similarly, when sitting down, she had to press on her knees to force them to bend.

Her physician assured me that there was no evidence of brain damage from the accident. Her case was a mystery to him. He asked whether the Alexander Technique helped with balance. On my assurance, he made the referral on behalf of the team of physicians that had worked with her. "We can't do anything more for her," he said.

After three lessons there was no response and I was ready to echo her doctor's words.

It was the woman's own perseverance that encouraged me. "I know these things take time," she said. "It's taken me four years to get this far. I'm going to continue lessons."

In this unique situation, I found that I had to change the way I normally work. Usually the Alexander student is asked *not* to think of doing the movement, not to think of bending the knees, of sitting down on a chair, or of standing up, but instead to think of the mental directions.

With her this did not work. I had to ask her to tell herself to sit down and stand up. I also added the Alexander directions. It worked. Gradually she improved. After some more lessons, I was able to drop the adaptation and then work only with the Alexander directions.

She started with me in April. During the cold of the next winter she reported that she had slipped on the ice three times but had not fallen. For a person who, a few months ago, fell at no provocation, this was a milestone. By this time, she was walking, sitting, and standing almost normally. She was functioning again at almost full capacity.

There are other extreme examples of medical problems that improve with Alexander lessons. Blood pressures go down. Headaches disappear. Gastro-intestinal disorders are alleviated. Bursitis and arthritis respond.

Women have come to a lesson with menstrual cramps and left 30 minutes later without them. Some, with chronic menstrual pain, are freed of this burden.

Alexander wrote of case histories involving the relief of asthma and of stuttering.

I have had cases of multiple sclerosis. They were not cured, but the Alexander lessons did provide relief from the varied symptoms that usually accompany that disease—pain in the legs, aching back, shaking, poor circulation, frequent urination, insomnia, weak reflexes, poor balance.

From the common cold to cancer, *stress* plays an important role, and the Alexander Technique is effective in releasing and preventing stress.

Recently, Stephen Locke of Boston University and McLean Hospital in Belmont, Mass. found that people who cope better with stress had a higher immune response. He exposed a sample of healthy blood to human leukemia cells. "Killer cells" attacked the leukemia which were tagged to release radioactive chromium. This activity was highest among those who showed fewest stress symptoms.

A woman with agonizingly painful rheumatoid arthritis since the age of 15 came to me for Alexander lessons. After her first half-hour lesson she reported that it was the first night in many years that she did not have insomnia. After two lessons she reported she no longer had headaches. After three lessons—all in the period of that first week—she reported she had *no pain*.

She continued for three weeks during which she was able to cut down her medication, including cortisone, by two-thirds. During this period she continued to be free of insomnia, headaches, and pain. She discontinued because her husband became quite ill but later resumed for reinforcement.

I have worked with people after hip and knee operations, as well as after spinal surgery, and helped them not only be relieved of their pain, but also to walk normally again. They learned to walk without a limp and to eliminate any poor effect on their alignment or balance that may have come about as a compensation.

People training their eyesight with the Bates Method of Vision Improvement have found that with the Alexander lessons they experience quicker vision improvement. In some cases, they break through a plateau to further improvement.

One does not have to take Alexander lessons for a prolonged period to find out whether or not it works. Improvement starts to take place almost immediately, usually during the first couple of lessons.

In some medical cases the consent of the physician is desirable. The physician should be informed, especially in cases of disc problems, that no exercises are performed in an Alexander lesson. Exercises are taboo for some severe disc problems. In my experience, once informed of the no-exercise aspect in such cases, physicians have readily given their consent.

Tension produces poor "use."

Poor "use" produces pain and disease.

Substitute proper "use" and its symptoms can wither on the vine and disappear as the good "use" takes over.

Maybe the calcium deposits or the damaged vertebrae remain, but their pain is diminished as the body tension diminishes, and pressure is relieved.

The Alexander Technique is not a treatment or a cure. It is an education. Whatever state your body is in, you learn to use it with the greatest positive results.

➡ Mental Health Problems Respond

Alexander teachers are receiving an increasing number of referrals from psychologists and psychiatrists as the acceptance grows of mind-body links.

One schizophrenic woman, who had been a patient in and out of mental hospitals for 20 years, was referred to me by her psychiatrist. Helen was a fairly attractive brunette in her mid-forties. She was not married now and was working on and off, depending on her mental state. Her present job was at a drugstore where it was understood that her attendance would be "iffy."

The referring psychiatrist had seen a demonstration of the Alexander Technique by me the previous week. Helen had just been referred to him by another psychiatrist, and after an initial examination he said he thought the Alexander training offered promise in Helen's case.

He gave me a brief history of how Helen had not been responding to psychiatric treatment. Only shock treatment seemed to be effective. "Alexander is worth a try," he said, "as an alternative to shock treatment."

Helen's body was jerky and clumsy. Her sister drove her over as she was not well enough to drive herself. She walked awkwardly. Her speech was halting and spasmodic. She went through the Alexander movements in a stiff manner. At the end of the half-hour period, I detected a slight lessening in this stiffness, but not much else.

When Helen returned for the second lesson, she told me that she had gone shopping with her sister after the first lesson. "We shopped for hours together. The time went so fast." This was good news, because this had been a low period when all she did was lie around at home. "And I drove myself here today," she said proudly.

As her lessons continued, Helen's body became more integrated. She walked and talked more smoothly. Her psychiatrist and I spoke on the telephone after each lesson, and I told him of some of the things Helen said during her lessons. He was amazed at these and said they would never have come out in psychiatric treatment. "This is like going around through the back door," he said.

Helen became more and more agile. She became active and alive. She was obviously reaching a higher level of well-being and happiness. After only six or seven lessons, her speech and body were normal, her intelligence shone through and one would never suspect what Helen had experienced.

Then something strange happened.

Helen began to engage me in long conversations before each lesson. She seemed to be stalling. One afternoon she sat down in the waiting room and did not want to go into the Alexander room. She engaged me in small talk for 20 minutes. The lesson is 30 minutes.

When I insisted on starting the lesson, she finally said, "You know I have improved so much in these Alexander lessons that I am now faced with having to consider relationships with men. It has been 20 years since I have had such a relationship. I don't know how to do it." With that she got up and left and never came back. She also never went back to the psychiatrist.

Helen was afraid of getting well. She was sane in that she recognized this; most people who protect their illness do so without ever knowing what they are doing.

➡ Institutional Applications

A psychiatric hospital on the West Coast sponsored a series of seminars on body-related therapies, and I was asked to participate. The seminar was for the hospital staff, and mental patients were brought in to each seminar to be worked on. I was invited to present the Alexander Technique, as the last in the series.

During my seminar I demonstrated on both a male and female psychiatrist; both of them were very rigid, and only one of them was slightly responsive. I worked approximately 20 minutes with each one.

They then brought in a mental patient, a woman of around 60; she had been in mental hospitals for the past fifteen years, I was told. She walked in as stiff as a block of wood. When I started to work with her, there was no response; she was more rigid than the two doctors. After about five minutes, as I continued working with her on the table, her muscles became softer and more pliable, her joints more flexible and her limbs more supple. The difference was quite re-markable.

After about fifteen minutes of table work, I brought her up off the table. Her face was radiant. She walked happily around the room several times as if she was showing off a new dress. "My muscles feel so free," she kept saying. "I love this."

She was brought back in the afternoon for a followup. This time I did Alexander work on the chair. After a brief demonstration, she stood up and fairly pranced around the room, exclaiming, "I feel so good. I feel so free. I'm rarin' to go. I want to go back to my job."

There was an audible gasp from the staff who knew her as a typist who had lost her desire to work and had become relatively immobile.

At the conclusion of the seminar, the staff agreed that only two therapies of those demonstrated had shown effectiveness: Rolfing and the Alexander Technique. There was a leaning in the direction of Alexander over Rolfing, as the Rolfing involved physical pain, which was not considered advisable for mental patients.

They decided to hire an Alexander teacher who would work first on the staff members themselves and then on the patients. They had noted that the families of mental patients were rigid people. The ones who were trying to help the mental patients should *not* be rigid. Ultimately, the Alexander teacher would train staff members to be teachers. It was a good idea and a sound approach.

I recommended an Alexander teacher, and the staff invited him to come for two days, for discussions. During that time he worked on three different mental patients, for a half hour each. A week later, the director sent us both reports informing us that one patient had been slightly improved, and the other two had shown remarkable changes: one of them, who was habitually very hostile to all those around him, had not made an unpleasant remark for two days afterwards; and the other, who had been in a wheelchair because of difficulty in walking, had been walking and not using his wheelchair for several days after his lesson. *And each one had had only one half hour of "Alexandering."*

These mental patients had shown a faster and more dramatic improvement in their behavior after one Alexander lesson than most other people. Everyone involved was very enthusiastic about the new project of including an Alexander teacher on their staff.

Unfortunately, the project did not come about. There was money available to hire another staff member; however, the hospital superintendent decided that the money would be better used to build another parking lot! The Director of Education for the hospital, who was the prime mover behind the seminars, resigned from his position in deep disappointment.

A western state prison for the criminally insane was also interested in hiring an Alexander teacher. The state was making special funds available for rehabilitation. The Chief Psychiatrist of the prison had read an article by a British penal superintendent endorsing the Alexander Technique. He wrote to me that according to this article, a system based on reward called operant-conditioning, which worked quite well in prisons, was far more effective when used in conjunction with Alexander lessons. Would I come and provide a demonstration of the Technique and a plan for implementation? I agreed to go there for a few days the following month. Not long after,

I received an almost tearful letter from the Chief Psychiatrist stating that the government's offer of funds had been withdrawn, to be used for other purposes.

A general statement I could make about the effect of the Alexander Technique on students referred by psychiatrists and psychologists, is that they respond better to their psychiatric or psychotherapy treatments. They open up and reveal their inner states more readily, and suddenly make rapid progress, often leading to an early discharge.

It is often agreed by the referring doctor that the improvements that come after the patient started Alexander lessons may not have come about at all without the lessons. It becomes evident that releasing the blocks in the body is a necessity for fuller change. The tensions and "armoring" of the body act as a prison, imprisoning a large degree of the freedom and joy within a person, which does not become unlocked through mental work alone. Wilhelm Reich was the first psychoanalyst to realize this, and he modified his therapy accordingly.

When treating people with the acknowledgement that body, mind and emotions are interconnected, far greater progress is made in helping people realize their full potential of health and well-being.

I have often found that students of the Technique who have also had some form of emotional therapy or psychotherapy respond faster, and possibly go further than those who have not. Working with body, mind and emotions is more complete than working with only one aspect.

Occasionally, as in the case of Helen, a person enjoys getting well at first, but cannot tolerate getting too close to normal. They begin to feel that they have social and sexual responsibilities that seem to be too threatening to them, and they discontinue their lessons.

Perhaps one answer is to maintain the in-patient status for such people during the process of reeducation, so that the impact of life is not a deterrent to progress. Life is interrelation of body, mind and spirit; thal also means dealing with money, sex, and other people.

Those who are too fearful to enjoy their renewed health are rare cases. Most people who take Alexander lessons joyfully absorb the improvements in their life.

Chapter 5

Meet Your Alexander Teacher— And Be Introduced To Nondoing

DOES THE ALEXANDER TEACHER demand hard work, effort, and repetitive homework practice? Is your teacher a person who says to you: "Stand up straight, shoulders back. Look how crookedly you walk with your feet; force your feet to be straight; force your legs to be straight. Hold your head up and straighten your back. Stand against a wall and press your back against the wall and *hold* that position as you walk."

The answer is no. The Alexander mind-body approach is quite the opposite of sweat, strain and effort. An Alexander teacher is likely to say: "If it hurts, don't do it." The teacher is kind and caring. This kind of teacher wants you to rediscover the easy, pleasurable way of moving. Your teacher embodies the Alexander approach.

"Any homework, teacher?"

"No."

"Shouldn't I practice getting in and out of a chair?"

"No, not even that."

There is one kind of home practice which many Alexander teachers find to be valuable. The student is asked to let the Alexander thoughts accompany the body in everyday movements. That is, one thinks in a light, easy way of the Alexander thoughts while moving through the day. This is the only discipline required, the discipline to remember to say: neck free, head forward and up, back lengthening and widening. Give yourself light, easy thoughts *instead* of trying to move right. Alexander usually insisted that people come to him five times a week. When going as frequently as that for lessons, there is not such a need for directing oneself in between lessons. Those who come for lessons only once or twice a week will also progress satisfactorily without directing in between lessons; with these people, though, the progress is speeded up significantly by frequent reminders in between lessons.

While walking, driving your car, or washing dishes, lightly direct your head to move forward and up and your back to lengthen. A slight lowering of the chin is helpful to release the neck and back muscles.

Some students, who feel so good during the lessons, want to extend them at home. "What can I do at home for myself?" is a frequent question. My answer: *"Lie down and do nothing."*

I elaborate by explaining that they are to lie on the floor with their knees up, legs and feet spread apart, one or two books under the head, and to give themselves the Alexander instructions.

This is exactly the same as what they do in the table work part of the lesson with the teacher. They can do this from five to fifteen minutes at a time. It often does wonders. After that, it is important to come up to standing gently so as not to tighten the back and spine. The easiest way is to slowly roll onto one side, on to the hands and knees, and slowly come to a standing position, leaving the head

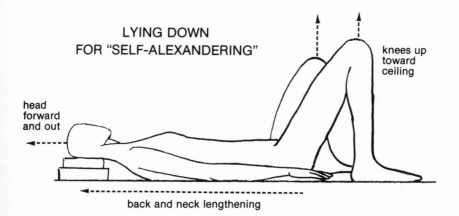

LYING DOWN
FOR "SELF-ALEXANDERING"

knees up
toward
ceiling

head
forward
and out

back and neck lengthening

lowered and looking down. At the very end allow your eyes to look at eye-level and let your head gently follow. We like to choose the easy way to do things. This "self-Alexandering" is also marvelous when tired. You come up feeling rejuvenated.

Your Alexander teacher is a person who shows you how to give up the struggle of getting through life. The Alexander teacher shows the way to bring ease into your life, and the joy of a new way of being.

➡ The Training of an Alexander Teacher

Who is this person who is guiding you in your thoughts and speaking to you with gentleness and understanding?

The Alexander teacher has gone through a long intensive training. The Alexander approach requires very subtle skills, and subtlety is acquired less readily than more forceful ways; it comes by way of a long and patient route.

There are currently several schools where an Alexander teacher candidate can go for training. There are three in the United States, all part of the American Center for the Alexander Technique: one in New York City, another in San Francisco, and the third in Chicago. From time to time there is a training program in Los Angeles.

There are training schools in London; three of them are headed by men who trained under F. Matthias Alexander himself—Wilfred Barlow, M.D., Walter Carrington and Patrick Macdonald. The British training schools are listed with the Society of Teachers of the Alexander Technique in London.

There are several Alexander teachers in Israel who trained in London, and now there is a training program in Jerusalem.

The period of training usually runs three years. Three years is a long time. Yet, this is what Alexander teachers have gone through to be able to sense with a gentle touch, and to establish communication in their unique way. Since the training is usually one-and-a-half to two-and-a-half hours daily five times a week, it is scheduled to accommodate part-time or fulltime occupations of those trainees who need to work while they train.

A Certificate is given at the end of the training period. If a trainee is considered not ready to teach at that time, he or she may continue their training for an additional period until ready to be certified.

Trainees are permitted to join a class at various times; in this way a training class includes beginners, intermediate and advanced trainees. When the class is structured this way, the advanced students can help the beginners, and progress is more rapid.

Entrance requirements vary. Some schools include a prerequisite of a period of Alexander lessons prior to entrance into the program. In schools where this is not a requirement, the new trainee is not permitted to work on anyone during the first months.

Trainees work on each other, as well as on the training teacher. In this way, trainees are daily being "Alexandered" and are constantly improving their own "use." This daily "Alexandering" and self-improvement is an essential part of the training.

An Alexander teacher cannot transmit good direction to another person unless he or she has excellent direction and good use for himself or herself. The touch of the Alexander teacher needs to be developed to encourage the lengthening of muscles in the person they are touching. Many people touch other people and cause them to "contract," which is a reaction of becoming tense from the touch. In fact, this is a frequent sequence. Touch. Contract. When you are touched by a person who is tense, the feeling of that touch is not as pleasant as that of a relaxed person who "has it together." This is perceptible in massage, or a simple handshake, or a pat on the back. The positive touch is essential in an Alexander teacher.

A major part of the training process is to release the tension in your own body, through being "Alexandered," and to learn how to maintain the freedom in your body (which we call "good direction") while working on someone else. Another aspect of the training is to learn to recognize what one feels with one's fingers or hands on another person.

➡ Nondoing

Alexander stressed "nondoing," and this is essential for both student and teacher. *Nondoing* encompasses NOT trying to do the action in the *right* way, and also NOT trying to *make* one's neck free or *make* one's head go forward and up or one's back to lengthen and widen.

An Alexander teacher has learned to apply *nondoing* while teaching, so that the teacher does NOT try to force the head and back of the student to go upwards, and also is NOT concerned with the activity they are working with, let us say standing up, but *instead* is giving the Alexander directions. The Alexander teacher directs himself or herself silently, while communicating the directions verbally to the student. The teacher has learned to recognize the response of upward "direction" in the student's body, and how to move the student effortlessly from one position to another (for example, from sitting to standing) while maintaining ease in their own body as well as in the student.

"Just how does this occur?" you may be wondering.

The student is sitting on a chair, and the teacher stands at the side of the chair facing the student. The teacher's hands are delicately touching the student's head and neck. The teacher directs himself silently and aloud asks the student to direct himself. When they both direct there is an instant response in the student of the head going up and the back lengthening. The student often thinks the teacher's hands have moved him. This is not so. The power of the combined direction has moved him. The student is now ready to carry out a physical movement with good use. The teacher continues to give his own directions and he allows his hands to float upwards; if the student continues to give *his* directions, he floats with the teacher's hands up to standing.

This does not at first always happen smoothly. At any instant the process can be sabotaged by either the student or the teacher *even thinking of doing the physical movement*. Usually it is the student. When this happens, the student's body contracts, and tension results. The teacher feels this instantly, and reminds the student to think of length.

Perhaps the most difficult part of the training is the NON-DOING. It is actually a *mental* discipline, and, as I have stressed before, the body follows the mind.

It requires a gread deal of training to move someone else *without thinking of moving them*, refraining from any effort on one's own part, and to *completely trust* the mental directions. An Alexander teacher has to apply to himself, while teaching another person, the same teaching that he is imparting to that person.

This teaching involves three concepts developed by Alexander: NONDOING, END-GAINING and MEANS WHEREBY. All three concepts are interrelated.

END-GAINING means being concerned with reaching your goal (or "end"). End-gaining is discouraged in the Alexander work. Psychologists today use the term "goal-oriented" for the same concept.

NONDOING—the act of *not* trying to do what feels right, and *not* thinking of the activity, allows you to substitute MEANS WHERE-BY for end-gaining.

For example, *as soon as you decide to stand up*, you are likely to go into a series of tense actions in your body to move out of the chair: shortening the back of your neck, pulling your head backwards and downwards, hunching your shoulders, and arching your back, and some people also bring their knees together. None of this is necessary to get out of a chair. Watch little children or a good actor and you will see they do not go through these contortions.

Instead, let us use NONDOING and MEANS WHEREBY. As soon as you decide to get out of the chair, you can say to yourself: "I am *not* going to think of getting out of the chair, I will *not try* to do it." You can then add: "Instead, I will lower my chin softly and tell my head it is floating forwards and upwards. I continue to tell my head to float forwards and upwards and my back to lengthen and widen as I allow my body to come up." This result, after a while, can be achieved with an abbreviation of the thoughts, eventually without the need to say anything, and finally, without a teacher.

Deciding *not* to try and stand up on the first instant is what Alexander called INHIBITION. This allows NONDOING to take place, and eliminates END-GAINING. You are left with MEANS WHEREBY—using the directions—and can reexperience your original good, natural use.

Instead of trying to *do* the right thing, and being involved in effort, NONDOING *undoes* the "efforting" you have developed over the years. Without that "efforting" you are left with effortless movement.

Your Alexander teacher has learned to apply this to himself, as well as to teach it to others, both verbally and through touch—a nondoing touch.

An Alexander teacher has been taught that *doing nothing* while touching another person *is better than doing the wrong thing*. And what we experience is that by simply touching, *while directing ourselves*, the "right" thing *happens*—it does *not* happen when we *try to do* the right thing.

▶ The Trainee Learns Good Use

Lulie Westfeldt had experience with teachers' training courses from February, 1931 to September, 1938, at 16 Ashley Place in London where Alexander trained his first teachers. She rates the conditions under which those trainees worked as "highly favorable." Alexander worked with them for two hours in the morning and the graduate teachers gave them additional help in the afternoon.

She said that many competent teachers were turned out in those days thanks largely to this extra help provided by then graduate teachers. About half of them stayed on to provide this assistance to Alexander. Later, two of the graduate teachers, Walter Carrington and Patrick Macdonald, became his chief assistants.

Lulie Westfeldt wrote in her book *F. Matthias Alexander: The Man and his Work** of the effects of the training program on the participants:

"In addition to the great physical improvements, most of them thought in a more organized way, with less confusion and greater consciousness. Some handled their lives with more mastery and ease; they lived more successfully and happily."

The training is a process of both receiving and of giving. By sheer repetition, the sensitivity of the trainee grows until fingertips become biofeedback devices.

As a trainee progresses, his or her own body is so in balance with good use that the obstacle of personal tension is removed. Freedom and openness is communicated through the hands. An Alexander teacher's hands are to be relaxed to encourage "lengthening," the opposite of "contraction." You feel the difference. Some people decided to take lessons simply from the way they were touched by a person who was an Alexander teacher.

The trainee is reminded constantly to direct himself or herself

*See Bibliography

while touching someone else. Proper use of the trainee's body is essential while teaching. So, for the teacher-trainee, self-direction is constantly going on. The good direction that the teacher's body enjoys is transmitted through the hands to the student.

This is the basic experience as the training proceeds, and continues with the graduate Alexander teacher. An experienced teacher no longer needs to constantly think of self-direction while teaching as he or she is well-directed all or most of the time.

➡️ Subtle Body Signals That Are Detected

During my first training sessions, my teacher placed her hands lightly on top of mine as I was touching someone else's head and neck.

Then all three of us—the subject, my teacher and myself—gave ourselves the directions, "Let the neck be free, to let the head go forward and up . . ."

After a moment, my teacher said. "Oh, now the length is coming through. Can you feel it, Judith?"

I could not feel a thing. I had thought I had sensitive hands, but time after time my teacher felt a reaction and I felt nothing.

When I returned home after that first time I asked my neighbor to permit me to practice on her what I had learned. What I had learned was touching *without doing*. She agreed. I gave the directions, and could feel no change, but she did. In fact, her frequent headaches disappeared from that day on and she was eager for me to continue to use her to practice what I learned each time.

It tooka few training sessions before I could feel any sensation at all. Then I began to detect the faintest "whisper" of change in the body.

The slight change that takes place in a body as a response to a thought is *very subtle*. The electromyograph picks it up easily, but the fingers do not, unless they go through repeated experiences and subtle training. Finally comes the dawn. The trainee's fingers are able to sense.

The sensations we detect vary. Sometimes we feel a current going through the body. Or we can actually feel a movement of the spine as it gets longer, or sense movement in the back as the back lengthens. In some cases the movement is obvious and you can easily *see* the lengthening in terms of a fraction of an inch or more. Even the casual observer can sometimes see the torso lengthen. At other times it is imperceptible, although easily felt.

Whether lengthening is subtle or pronounced, it is always an *involuntary* movement. The person is *not pulling* himself more erect, it *happens* from the thoughts contained in the directions.

One young actor to whom I gave Alexander lessons was interested in feeling this subtle lengthening. I asked him to lightly hold my arm as I gave my neck-head-back directions. Although he could not see anything happen, he could feel it. He was very excited by the sensation of lengthening. "Like pulling the lobster meat out of the claw," was the way he described the feeling. The lengthening *from the inside* is quite different from the forced stretching of an arm. It goes further. There is actually *more* stretch, in a gentle, natural way.

Detecting subtle changes of the body and learning to interpret them is an essential part of the training. This comes with the development of constant direction in oneself and of an exquisite sensitivity in one's fingers.

It takes a lot of practice. While moving a student it is very easy to tighten oneself and forget one's own directions. As soon as one *even thinks* of trying to move a student, there is contraction. It takes place in both the teacher and the student. In this sense, the teacher does no more than an advanced Alexander student, focusing on his own length while moving. The teacher, however, is also moving another person, and has to refrain from thinking of his own movement as well as refrain from thinking of moving the student. Instead, the movement "happens" while thinking the Alexander directions.

➡ The Excitement of Learning

You may wonder how a trainee can survive month after month of repetitive training.

There is always the excitement of feeling the person's body respond under your hands with greater lengthening, fluidity, lightness and ease. These are constant, pleasurable "rewards." There is the excitement of feeling this response first in one activity, then in another: "Today, I began to take my subject up out of a chair!"

With each movement there is the starting over again of the process of not trying, and of directing oneself as well as the person. When the movement is effortless, easy and fluid, one is ready to go on to another movement. Sitting. Standing. Walking. Going into a squat. Bending. Up and down on the toes. Reaching up with the arms. Reaching sideways. Turning the body at different angles. Moving the head in different directions.

Eventually, one can work with *any* movement, and feel the delicious quality of another person's body yielding and flowing with the movement.

The joy of life in the body.

➡ In the Field

A good Alexander teacher will invent thoughts which apply to different parts of the body and to different activities. This is totally in keeping with the Alexander process. We learn to extrapolate, adapt and extend, beyond Alexander's directions.

For instance, I asked one pianist to think of her fingers and wrists as putty, in addition to directing "lengthening." This instantly relaxed her tense hands. Saying "Neck free, head forward and up, back lengthening," had not been sufficient to counteract her *additional* tension at the piano.

Once you understand the mind-body relationship, you also understand that helpful thoughts can vary. One needs to be careful to choose words that lead to more lightness and ease. Some thoughts lead to more lightness than others. For instance, the concept of putty is a lighter thought than the use of the word clay. Creating a hole in the wall to permit the bedridden musician's head to extend out is easier than moving a wall backward. I often use a variation that is just as effective as a hole in the wall—that there is no wall there at all. The thoughts can be various and varied. *The essence of the work is to use thought, to let the mind direct the body.*

You, too, can be inventive in your thoughts as you do the movements that we share in this book, and also as you do the movements of your daily life. Mental thoughts that contribute to the ease of motion are *all* valid.

Which is a better thought—floating in water or floating in space? Whichever you prefer is the better one. There can be times when one will work better than the other and the reverse can also happen.

However, the neck, head and back thoughts are the essence. Any added thoughts are an extension to specific body parts and to the specialized motions of those parts to increase effectiveness.

Let us say you have decided to give yourself Alexander directions as you walk across the room. You walk across the room, imagining that your neck is free so that your head can go forward and up to permit your back to lengthen and widen.

It is an easy walk. You may feel slightly unnatural with something new, but you feel a greater ease in walking. You resolve to give yourself these directions the next time you walk out of the house. It so happens, the next time you remember to do this is an hour later when you walk the dog.

Now you have a new situation. The dog is jumping all over you as you walk toward the front door. Once outside there is a constant tugging on the leash by the dog, or you must tug on the leash when the dog stops to sniff at every tree.

How do you give yourself directions now? What do you think as you pull the dog forward or back? How do you enhance the use of your body?

Can you think of an elastic leash? How about an elastic arm that lengthens, all the while thinking of lengthening upwards. Can you conceive of the whole procedure as a lengthening dance with the dog as your partner? These concepts can turn a stressful tug-of-war into a stressless caper.

These are the kinds of concepts that the Alexander teacher needs to be capable of inventing for specific situations.

Alexander himself "ad-libbed" and some of the innovations found their way into the training, in addition to the neck-head-back directions and the movements of sitting, standing, walking, and bending. Some teachers who trained with Alexander himself were given movements and directions that were not part of the training for earlier students.

When a student is "stuck," it takes skillful use of words by the teacher, as well as skillful hands, to bring the student out of the dark and into the light. Occasionally, a student who is taking lessons with me gets "stuck." An impasse is reached. I must come up with a new thought which gets the student on a different mental track. This is part of the Alexander Technique.

I believe this is an important part of the Alexander teacher-training. During the three years of training you learn how to direct a person through an impasse through innovating new thoughts. In the field, it is often necessary.

➡ Ups and Downs During the Training

There were many times during my training that I became discouraged, even despondent.

"I was never cut out to be an Alexander teacher," I would say. "I ought to drop the whole thing."

But then would come a moment of "Ah hah!"

These "Ah hah!" experiences kept me going.

"Ah hah! This is what my trainer has been talking about all these months."

I finally felt it! Another subtle sensing crossed the threshold of consciousness.

"Let me feel that again!"

The thrill is hard to describe. The body under your hands has communicated no response time after time. "There. Can't you feel that?" "No, I must say I didn't feel a thing." It is very discouraging. Then, one day the body under my fingertips moved ever so slightly. Like a feather, or as if it was levitating. Ah hah!

Even after the years of training are over and the trainee has become a teacher, "Ah-hah!" experiences continue to feed the thrill of teaching. I have that thrill to this day, even after sixteen years of teaching!

Being out on one's own in the world, dealing with bodies that you have never experienced before is rather different than being in the training program. Sometimes the bodies do not respond well. This brings back those memories of discouragement as a trainee. You innovate, you adapt, you expand your expertise, and along comes the moment of "Ah hah!"

It can make you want to dance a jig.

➡ The Teacher's Touch

In the training sessions, the teacher-trainee is taught to use a gentle touch which tends to "lengthen" and lighten the subject, whereas a harsh touch would "contract" the subject.

Sometimes a firmer touch is called for. With experience, a teacher learns how to use a firmer touch in a way that "lengthens," and will occasionally use a firm touch without sacrifice of extension. This firmer touch is not a massage, nor is it coercion. It merely gives a "louder" message with the hands. However, the "Alexander" touch is usually light, gentle and "nondoing," bringing about rather remarkable changes that usually cannot be achieved with a heavier touch.

I am going to ask you to experience the different effects of a light and heavy touch, but first I want to say that when you are directing with your mind for extension (neck free, head forward and up, back lengthening and widening) a hard touch has less chance of contracting you.

Here is a way to feel a difference in touch:

Clasp your hands firmly with fingers interlocked. See how that feels. Now let go. See what the after-effect is like. Shake your hands gently a few times to rid yourself of the effect. Wait a few seconds.

Now proceed to place your hands in a position to repeat this clasp but do not yet permit them to touch. Lightly intertwine your fingers. Do not clasp them, just permit the sides of the fingers to touch ever so gently with a soft touch of your fingertips on the backs of your hands. When I do this, I feel a tingling. Perhaps you do, too.

Now slowly separate your hands. Can you still feel the effects on the fingers? The touch seems to linger. Perhaps the tingling lingers. If you are not sure, do it again.

The gentle touch has many ramifications, many facets, and they seem to echo and reecho; the touch lingers.

Let us do something different.

Very gently grasp your left wrist with your right hand, slightly above your left hand. Pretend that you are not grasping your wrist but instead you are gently holding a baby bird. Did your touch change with that thought? Did it become lighter?

Be your left wrist. How does it feel, left wrist, to be held gently as if you were a baby bird? Do you feel the warmth? The caring?

Remove your right hand. Be aware of the after-effects.

It is as if the love of the mother bird has unmistakably left its mark.

If you wish, you could experience a contrast. Grasp your left wrist again. Tighten this grasp. Make it firm.

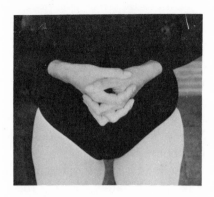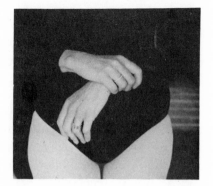

Now be your left wrist. How do you feel, left wrist? Presumably, not too comfortable. Let go. Notice the after-feeling. Shake your hands out to free the hand and wrist.

If I were to touch your left wrist as an Alexander teacher, the contrast you felt between firm and gentle would be greater and the after-effects would be likewise more pronounced.

The teacher is trained to such a subtle degree that it seems at times that he or she is reading the student's mind through touch.

➡ The Difference Between Directed
and Nondirected Movement

Stand up with your feet together. Now separate your feet by about twelve inches by gently stepping to one side with one foot (not shuffling). What did you do with your body to step to one side with that foot?

Probably, you first thought of the foot with which you would step sideways; then you placed your weight on the other foot and stepped to one side quite heavily with the first foot, shifting your weight from one foot to the other.

The Alexander teacher does not want it to happen this way. What the Alexander teacher wants you to be thinking of is not which foot to move or how to move it (which is *end-gaining*) but—yes, you guessed it—neck free, head forward and up, back lengthening and widening (this is *means whereby*). *Think of your weight going upwards* as you step to one side, instead of your weight going from one side to the other, this eases the movement. There is a softness about the motion as the decision to move is eclipsed by these other thoughts. The basic lengthening directions allow *all* parts of the body to move more freely and lightly, all the way to the toes. Try it again.

Stand. Begin thinking *lightly* of your neck being free, of your head moving forward and up, and of your back lengthening and widening and of your weight going upwards. Now let one foot step to one side any time you wish, *while* repeating the thoughts.

That may have felt different to you. It would have felt different to the Alexander teacher. The teacher is able to detect whether the thoughts are on the neck, head and back or on the movement. An experienced teacher can sense this even *without* touching the person.

We learn to "read" what the student is thinking when moving. Sometimes, in the middle of a movement, a person will tighten. We not only recognize it instantly, we seem to be able to know just which thought caused it, just as we know when a person is thinking of "lengthening."

It goes beyond touch.

➤ Teachers See Through Clothes

Student keep their clothing on during the lessons, and teachers are trained to look at bodies and see through the clothing. Postural defects are noticed. Teachers can see what is crooked, what is straight, and what is out of alignment.

Of course, it is easy, clothing notwithstanding, to see if a person has one shoulder higher than another. But less obvious matters can be seen, too, such as contracted muscles. We can see through a loose jacket whether one hip is higher than another and we can determine through a pants leg whether one leg is more tense than the other.

How does a trainee acquire this ability? Different trainers may have different ways. In my training program, I have the trainee look, and look, and look.

I tell my trainees to look at a "body," while the "body" stands in front of a mirror. Regardless of whether the "body" is a trainee or not, I want him or her to also see what we are looking at.

The trainees are then asked to detect what is out of alignment, what is not level, what is different on one side of the body than the other side, from head to toe. Then I add my own observations. We do the same with the profile.

As time goes on, the trainees begin to see more and more. The eye becomes trained to seek out misalignment, imbalance, and tensions. This is also a good procedure for students to get to know their bodies. Use your mirror to discover your own body.

As the trainee progresses, he learns to pick up clues to body tension from movements like standing up, sitting down, and walking, as well as from standing still. We also learn to recognize *good use* and *good alignment* through clothes.

We need to give Alexander credit for developing this ability to see through clothes. Living, as he did, in the Victorian era, necessity was the mother of his invention. Even medical people in those days did not ask people to undress. Hence, our "x-ray" vision.

➡ The Trainee Becomes an Alexander Teacher

When the trainee completes the three-year stint, the world is his. He or she is an independent teacher. The length and frequency of the lessons are up to the teacher. It is at the discretion of the new teacher to set his own fees.

A new teacher usually gives a 45-minute lesson. As teachers become more experienced, they often reduce the lesson to 30 minutes. A very experienced teacher can teach more in thirty minutes than a new teacher can in 45 minutes. The fee varies according to talent and experience.

Teachers vary in personality, and also, to some extent, in their approach. Some teachers communicate a great deal verbally, others prefer to work mostly in silence. Some teachers prefer to start the lesson with chair work, others with table work. Some will work primarily with sitting and standing and bending, while others will work with a greater variety of movements. Some do very little movement during a lesson, focusing almost exclusively on the lengthening that comes through the directions, and others like to actively move a student frequently during a lesson.

Students also vary. Some prefer one type of teacher, some another. Some like to learn from only one teacher, others prefer to go to more than one teacher, either at the same time or at different times.

Some take lessons at an intense rate over a shorter period of time, while others spread the lessons over a longer period of time. Some students, after a significant period of lessons, discontinue permanently. Some students, after discontinuing lessons, like to come for a refresher of a few lessons once a year or so, and others prefer to continue for years on a non-intensive basis anywhere from once a week to once a month.

My first months as an Alexander teacher were, in a way, an extension of the "Ah-hah!" experiences of my training days. During the training period we trainees had become aware not only of the bodies of our fellow trainees, but also of those of people in the street. We were seeing through their clothing and thinking, "What I could do for that back!" or "That neck!"

We had an "itch" to do corrective work for everyone. We found it quite frustrating. We had to restrain ourselves from putting our hands on any person's neck and back to show them a way out of their body misery. This continued into my early days as a teacher. It took awhile for me to realize that I cannot go about relieving the misalignment of all humanity. After some time, I settled down to the gratification of helping those who came to see me.

➡ Finding an Alexander Teacher

If you have decided that Alexander lessons are for you, you may or may not find a teacher in your area.

In the time since Alexander started training other teachers, less than fifty years have passed, and there have not been many "generations" of three-year training periods.

There are probably fewer than 500 working Alexander teachers in all the world today, with perhaps about 200 in the United States.

An Alexander Center may be listed in your phone book under "Alexander Technique" or under "American Center for the Alexander Technique, Inc." If there is no such listing, write to the closest Alexander Center to you for names in your area (see Appendix I).

Some teachers are more popular than others because of personality or method. If you are fortunate enough to have a choice in your city or town, you may want to meet more than one of them.

Alexander Centers refer only *certified teachers*. If you locate a teacher yourself, you would be wise to inquire from an Alexander Center about his or her qualifications. A person who sets himself or herself up as an Alexander teacher without the recognized training and certification, may do you harm through lack of knowledge and expertise.

Alexander teachers have spent three years in training. This is a large investment in time and money. Some go back for refresher courses at additional cost. This should be taken into consideration when you evaluate fees charged. To some people, the fees seem reasonable, to others they seem high. Most students of the Technique find that the lessons are worth every penny. They learn something invaluable that they could not learn anywhere else, achieving "what had before seemed impossible."* And to those in pain and on medication, who have gone from doctor to doctor, and from one esoteric practice to another, the relief is priceless. It is an investment that pays off in terms of *your life*.

Students are usually asked to take lessons at least twice a week, and more often if possible. People with severe disabilities require more frequent lessons. As the Alexander Technique is teaching people to change their habits, greater frequency of lessons is desirable, particularly at the start. In this way, there is less time in between lessons to allow the tense, contracted habits to return, and the foundation of good use is more solid.

Although it takes several weeks or months of lessons to reach a high level of reeducation it does not take long to begin to feel the benefits.

The benefits are noticeable after one or two lessons. That is only the beginning. The benefits accrue and accumulate. Students often forget, after a while, how they *used* to feel. *The changes stay with you*. The reeducation is a rediscovery of the freedom of your body and your whole being. You rediscover this hand-in-hand with your Alexander teacher. You are not alone. You are with someone who has taken that path and can show you the way.

When you recapture it, you float through life.

News Chronicle, "He Teaches The Way Back to Health," February 26, 1953.

Chapter 6

Joyous Discoveries You Make

I WOULD LIKE TO SUGGEST that you stand in front of a full-length mirror and look at yourself.

Look at your face. Observe your shoulders, your neck, your chest, your hips, your thighs, your knees, your calves, and look down at your feet.

Is your head tilted to one side? Is your neck straight or crooked? Are your shoulders level or not? Is your chest sunken, or is it protruding, or neither? Are your hips level, or is one higher than the other? Are your knees pressed against one another, or lightly touching, or far apart? Notice the rotation of your thighs; are they inwards or outwards? Are your calves straight, or are they curved sideways or backwards? Do your feet point straight ahead, or are they turning inwards or outwards?

Look at your face, observe it carefully, also your eyes. How are you breathing? Were you holding your breath or were you breathing normally?

Remember what you see in the mirror.

How do you feel right now? It is a good idea to write this down, as I am going to ask you later to rate yourself twice again.

Rate yourself from one to ten on each of these conditions: energy level; freedom from body malease; general well-being.

Now stand up again. Tighten the back of your neck and hunch your shoulders in an unnatural position and walk around the room like this for a few minutes. Straighten a pillow, pick up the telephone for an imaginary call, do anything else you can think of.

Keeping your neck tight and your shoulders hunched up, rate yourself again on how you feel. You are bound to have lost a few points in all three categories. Now restore your shoulders and neck to their natural position.

Just as you lose points for poor use, you gain points for good use and in a moment I will invite you to experience an improvement and rate yourself again.

"Liberating your body will give you a sense of joy," state Emily Coleman and Betty Edwards in their book, *Body Liberation.**

People who have taken Alexander lessons are not only able to cope better with life's needs, they rediscover the joy of having a body.

Whatever they do feels so much more pleasurable. This kind of pleasure raises to immeasurable peaks the joy of sufficient energy and freedom from pain or discomfort.

I have heard these peaks of pleasure described in various ways by people whose belief is actually stretched by what they feel as it transcends the way they felt before.

"I feel intoxicated." "People are captivated by me now and I seem to charm them." "It is like going from constant pain to constant ecstasy." "I am floating." "I feel born again." "I'm a new person!"

Students become elated, transported, jubilant. They wallow, revel, and luxuriate in their new-found "euphoria." To hear them, you would think them a pack of hedonists. One of my New York students in her fifties said: "When I left your place and went into the street, I felt as if I could throw my leg over the lampost!"

They are reacting to a new awareness that comes from a liberated body. Soon, they take their "heaven" for granted and the boisterous enthusiasm dies down. But the joy remains, as the good use remains. The feeling of upwardness, lightness and ease induced by the Alexander lessons is long-lasting.

Little wonder that some 50 years ago John Dewey recommended that public schools should teach the Alexander method.

*J.P. Tarcher, Los Angeles, CA, 1977.

The Contribution of
Body Awareness to Joy

Are you ready now to experience a taste of this joy? Then participate in the following exercise. When you have completed it, rate yourself once more on energy level, freedom from body malease, and general well-being.

Lie on your back on the floor, arms by your sides, palms down, your feet apart, approximately the same distance as the width of your shoulders. Sense how the various parts of your body lie on the floor: your back, your shoulder blades, your head, your arms and hands, your hips, the backs of your thighs, backs of your knees, your calves, and your heels. Breathe normally as your mind travels along your body.

Next, you will bend your knees in a different way than before. Slowly slide the outside edges of both feet up the floor until your heels are close to your body, and they cannot go any further.

Raise your feet off the floor by permitting your bent knees to float into the air and to hang over your body. Your feet are apart.

Linger in this position. Think of it as a resting position. Notice how your back sinks into the floor, how it releases and flattens. Breathe normally. Give yourself time to enjoy this baby-like repose. Wait for at least three breaths to pass. You may stay like this as long as you like.

I want to show you now a way to return your feet to the floor so that you maintain the restfulness you have just gained. *Slowly* let both your heels descend until they gently meet the floor, then let them slide *slowly* down the floor and apart from each other until your legs are once again extended along the floor, with feet apart.

If you have found this pleasurable repeat it a few times slowly.

A variation of resting on your back with your knees hanging over your body, is to stay in this position and cross your ankles. (See photos). See if you can sense an additional slight release in your back when you cross your ankles. Put a hand around each knee, and move your knees slightly up and down. Do very small movements, and notice how this releases your back. To lower your legs, slowly

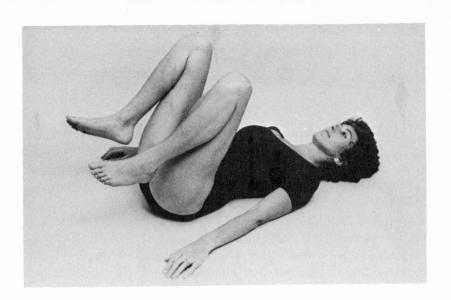

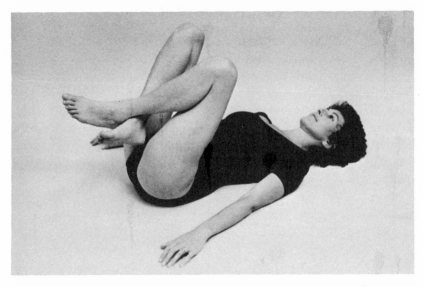

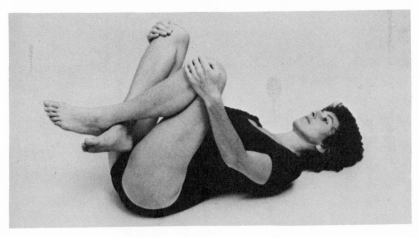

uncross your ankles and proceed to lower your feet and legs as before.

I invite you now to experience a series of movements that can give you more pleasurable feelings in your body and also add to your awareness.

Slowly slide your feet close to your buttocks and gently allow them to lift off the floor, and your knees hang over your body. Spread your arms out at shoulder level, palms up. Turn your head and look at your arms and see if each one is really at shoulder level. If you are surprised to see them either below or above shoulder level, this indicates that you are not clear about how your body moves and that your body may have certain "ways" about it that escape you. Most of us do not have a clear sense of awareness of ourselves.

With arms at shoulder level, move only your forearms, bending your arms at the elbows and bringing your hands to lie on each side of your head, backs of the hands against the floor.

You are now going to gently fold yourself over onto your right side. Move slowly in the way I describe, one movement after the other. Start by slowly moving your right knee to the right side, leaving it bent. Now let the left knee slowly follow and lie on top of it. Slowly your left arm is brought over to lie on top of your right arm, leaving the elbows bent at a 90° angle. Your knees also remain bent at a 90° angle.

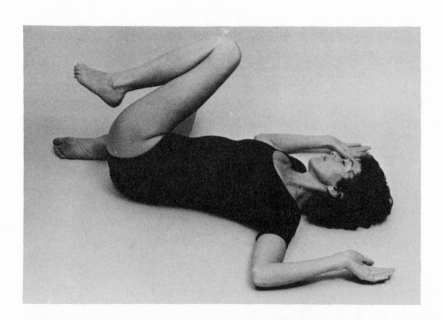

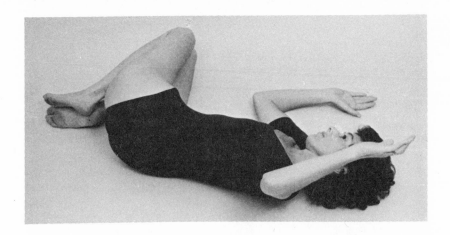

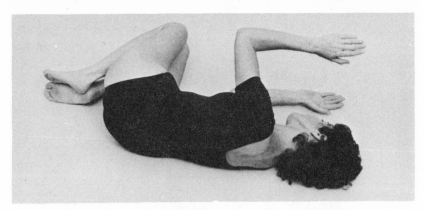

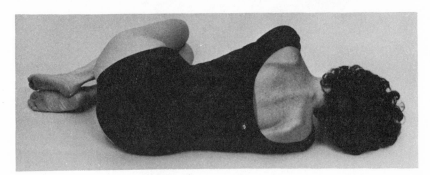

You are now lying "folded" together on the right side. Your left palm is on top of your right palm; your left elbow is on top of your right elbow; your left knee on top of your right knee and your left ankle and foot on top of your right ankle and foot.

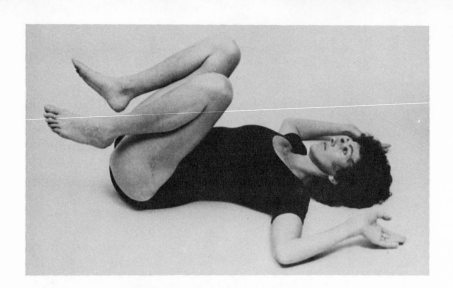

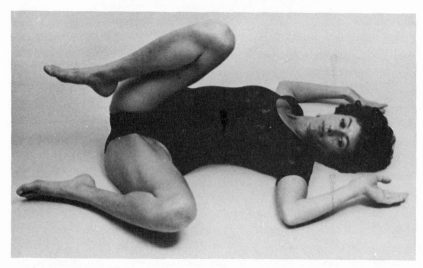

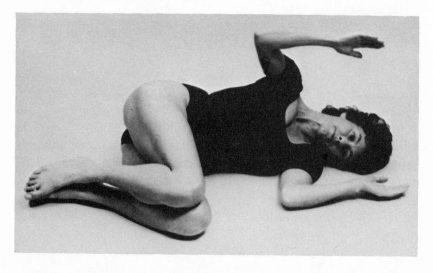

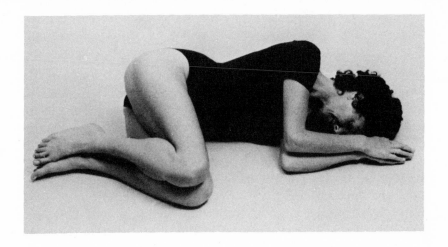

Feel how neat this "package" is. Savor it. Linger in it. Notice how soft your breathing is, how soft are your chest and belly. Feel how serene you are.

When you are ready to move, fold yourself to the other side by moving first the left arm gently to the floor on the left side, and then the left leg to the floor on the left side. Then slowly allow your right leg to follow the left, and finally let your right arm floatingly come to rest on top of the left arm.

Savor this left side "folded" position.

How does this side compare with the other side? Does one feel more cozy than the other? Does one side feel more familiar than the other?

When you are ready to move again, *slowly* fold yourself on to your right side: right arm first, then right leg, then left leg, and finally left arm.

Roll from side to side in this way, moving the limbs slowly and gently as if they are floating in the air. Breathe normally.

As your legs follow one another, floating through the air, your feet are apart. On the side, your feet are together.

As you go through the middle of each roll, you are opening up, and as your reach each side your are folded together. You go from folding to opening, from opening to folding, like the wings of a butterfly.

In this way, you are experiencing two different aspects of life. When folded on the side, you are protecting yourself, you are snug and secure and give yourself warmth and comfort. When opening up in the middle, you are allowing yourself to be vulnerable, you are receptive and open to what is around you. Some people's personalities are one-sided, either too closed and protective or too open and vulnerable. Both are necessary for us, and are appropriate at different times. Through these movements you can experience both, and allow yourself to go from one to the other at will.

When this movement becomes familiar to you, gradually increase the tempo. Always follow with one limb after the other, just as you did at the slower pace.

Be playful like a little child. Notice how your head rolls. Be aware how your whole body cooperates in the playful rhythm. Now go faster . . . faster and faster. Have fun with this. How fast can you go?

Gradually slow down, and sense another kind of joy in the slowing down. Gradually come to a halt, lying on your back. Lower your legs softly and slowly as you did before, heels meet the floor first, then they slowly slide down the floor and away from each other. Rest.

Lightly, let your mind skim over your body. Does it lie differently than before? Do some parts lie more easily on the floor? Let your mind travel gently over all parts of your body, from your head to your heels. Compare how you lie now with how you were lying *before* the movements. Observe your lower back, shoulder blades, head, arms and hands, hips, legs, and heels.

Slowly bend your knees one at a time, feet resting on the floor. Gently roll over onto your right side, with bent knees, then onto your hands and knees and up to a standing position. Do you feel different when standing? Walk around the room, in a natural way (*not* carefully). Does your body have a new buoyancy to it? Or a new ease? A new alignment? Where are your business anxieties or time pressures? Do you have a greater sense of aliveness and joy in your body now? Of relaxation? Of body awareness? Now score yourself on energy, freedom from malease, and level of well-being.

Look in the mirror to see if your body *looks* different. Observe all the parts, from your head to your toes. Look at your face. Is it more relaxed and happier? And your eyes, are they softer, more glowing?

Instructions for movements are lengthy. You can put the book down after reading the first instructions, then later pick it up for the next instructions. Or, you can have someone read you through it, or, best of all, *give yourself taped instructions.*

This is *not* the Alexander Technique. It is one of a number of series of movements developed by Dr. Feldenkrais that lead to the delicious changes that can take place when a gentle body-mind procedure is followed.

You may ask: "How was the mind involved?" Read the instructions again, and you will see that I was constantly asking you to think thoughts while moving, and to be aware of *how* you were moving. Instead of moving your limbs mechanically, like a machine, you moved softly following your thoughts.

A body-mind approach uses thoughts and awareness while moving the body, and results in a mental and emotional expansion that comes simultaneously with the freeing of your body.

The awareness of yourself that is developing is very important. How can you recognize poor habits and tension when you have not known anything different?

When tension is constant, it is not recognizable as tension. You may eventually feel the aches and pains that result from it, but the actual poor habits that involve the tension are below your awareness. Once you have experienced some release from the tension and know what greater freedom and better use feel like, then you are able to recognize the tension. In her article on the Alexander Technique,* Judith Leibowitz wrote: "The repeated experience of the new use creates an internal guide, a kinesthetic standard against which he now can measure himself... *only when the student has felt and recognized in his own body the correct usage can he feel and know the incorrect.* (Italics are mine.)

"Using this technique, one can consciously erase what was formerly automatic, habitual use, and, just as consciously, replace that habit with a better one until the new way itself becomes automatic."

▶ Alexander Lessons That Lead to Body Joy

Instead of exercises like the one you just enjoyed, the Alexander teacher leads you through the movements of your everyday life. These can include movements in addition to standing, sitting, walking, bending and lying down.

---

*"For the Victims of Our Culture: The Alexander Technique" by Judith Leibowitz, *Dance Scope*, Fall, 1969, Vol. 4 Number 1.

A tennis player might want to increase body awareness, and therefore the skill and joy of the sport, by having the Alexander teacher lead him through the simulated movements of serving, hitting a forehand drive or a backhand shot, retrieving a lob, or putting the ball away with an overhead smash. All are done to the "tune" of mental directions to let the neck be free, to let the head go forward and up, to permit the back to lengthen and widen. Or, in short, "lengthening." The teacher can see where the tennis player is over-contracting (or tensing) in these movements, and can direct additional directions to those specific areas.

(A tennis pro came for lessons after injuring his back twice. After standard Alexander directions to restore proper use, we worked on his serve and other strokes. I could see each instant he contracted. I then focused the directions for experiencing lengthening all the way through each stroke. It took care of everything and made him say, "You are my tennis teacher.")

The same advantages can be enjoyed by the golf player, bowler, bicyclist, jogger, and most certainly baseball, football and basketball players. It is important to eliminate "end-gaining," to give up thinking of your goal, whether it be hitting a tennis ball or a golf ball, and substitute "means whereby," using thoughts of lengthening *before* and *while* you allow your body to go through the motions of the movement, *instead* of thinking of the movement. IT IS HOW YOU THINK THAT COUNTS. *Think of your length instead of the goal.*

The same is true for dancers, musicians, weavers, potters, artists, writers, and fishermen. No matter what your sport, hobby or occupation, there are typical movements involved. These typical movements, when freed of tensions and misuse through Alexander directions, can be more enjoyable and more successful.

I often add additional thoughts for different activities and different people, but they are almost useless without the basic lengthening.

Emily, in her sixties, came for Alexander lessons with no special complaint. She had read about the Alexander Technique and wanted to get more joy out of her body and out of life. She enjoyed her lessons enormously. Then one day she told me how she played golf three times a week and was now taking golf lessons to improve her game. "The pro complains that I do not move my hips properly when I swing the club. Can you help?"

We went through a simulated stance and drive. I saw immediately what she was doing that was twisting her body into an unnatural alignment. Because she already had experienced the beneficial effects of the Alexander directions in other movements, it was a simple matter to have her use the same directions while driving a golf ball, with her body moving in a free-flowing way. This automatically eliminated her unnatural twisting of the hips.

She applied this on the golf course with a real golf club in her hands and told me when she returned that her golf pro had actually applauded her, exclaiming, "That's the way I've been trying to get you to move!"

A ballet dancer may say, "Well, it could not apply to the pirouette or other ballet movements. These depend on the dynamics of motion." It is those very dynamics that cry for proper use. Without it you have the shimmy of an unbalanced front tire which eventually can shake a car's body apart.

Whatever kind of dancer you are—ballet, modern, jazz—your Alexander teacher can show you how to apply the technique. Once applied, any movement of the body benefits.

This year, *Dance Scope* printed an article entitled "The Alexander Technique Gets Its Directions" by James H. Bierman. This article makes mention that the Alexander Technique was taught by Missy Vineyard at the 1978 American Dance Festival. Peggy Hackney, who works with the Bill Evans Dance Company, is quoted as saying about her experience with the Alexander Technique: "I was able to use my mind and awareness to help me progress faster. I wouldn't have made it where I am without the use of my mind." Deborah Caplan, an Alexander teacher in New York City, is a former dancer, and the article writes of her "having a similar edge during her years as a member of Jean Erdman's dance company as a result of her extensive experience with the Alexander Technique as a child. She was able to use the Alexander directions to be aligned and centered and to minimize the tendency to strain. They gave her a sense of connectedness and integration which most dance techniques lose in the emphasis on the articulation of parts. Like many other dancers who are familiar with the Alexander Technique, Deborah found the directions were of enormous help in warming up, and in the movement itself."

The article goes on to say: "The Alexander Technique enables students to move with responsibility by making them aware that they have a choice as to how to use their bodies rather than functioning automatically as an expression of accumulated habits. With this responsibility comes an enormous freedom. Pamela Anderson speaks eloquently of that freedom. 'Doing this work has given me the joy of movement again which I had lost in my striving to be technically perfect.' "

Do you sail a boat? You will sail faster as your movements become more harmonious. You will feel yourself synchronize with the breeze.

Do you assemble parts in a manufacturing company? You will flow with the assembly line as if you were part of it instead of intimidated by it.

Do you wash dishes, scrub and vacuum? It will be transformed from a chore to a "dance" as your body leads you through the movements rhythmically and effortlessly.

Holding a baby, chopping wood, shoveling snow, gardening: all require special movements. Because of the personality of the person, the movement is entered into with varying degrees of "mannerism" which, by definition, is something different from the normal.

Anything different from the normal places a strain on the body. If a jack is not in its normal position when you want to change a tire, something abnormal is going to happen. With the human body this abnormality can be a subtle tension. These tensions, when repeated, become not-so-subtle troubles.

Bettina, a cellist, found new joy in playing the cello. A slender, fairly attractive girl of 19, Betinna walked as if her body was cramped together. She looked pathetic. She was stoop-shouldered, sway-backed, and she seemed to be squashing down the whole of her right side.

After her first few Alexander lessons, her body became noticeably improved. I asked her to bring her cello in so that we could apply the Alexander Technique while playing. She brought her instrument with her at the next lesson and I asked for a recital. As soon as she had positioned herself and the cello and was ready to play, I stopped her.

"Bettina, as long as you place the instrument that way, you are forced to cramp your body." I sat down and imitated her posture. "See how I am cramping my body on the right side and hunching my shoulders over? How can my neck be free and how can my head go up and my back lengthen and widen?"

"But, that is the way I learned . . ."

I interrupted her because I had heard that story before. "That is the way your learned to tighten the right side of your body, hunch your shoulders, and curve your spine."

I adjusted the cello a little higher. She had had it too low, and had had to stoop down. She also had the cello at an angle which forced her to pull her left shoulder forward and around in order to finger the cello and, in the process, she had to pull her right shoulder backwards and pull down on her right side to use the bow. We changed the angle of the cello so that it was parallel to her body. This avoided her having to push one side of her body forward to play, and the other side backwards.

Bettina went along with these changes quite readily. Although she was playing in a position different from her previous experience, she found it comfortable and pleasurable. In this new position she could maintain her neck being free, her shoulders going out, and her head and back going up. She was pleased.

Then I noticed that the way she fingered with her left hand caused tension in her left shoulder, arm and wrist. The Alexander teacher can see tension across the room. Hers was obvious to me but she was oblivious to it herself. It took only a slightly different angle of contact with the strings to release the tension in her left hand and arm.

She objected to this. "No, I can't do that. These parts of the cushions of the fingers *must* be in contact with the strings."

She was a student of Claus Adams, one of the finest cellists in New York and a member of the Juilliard Quartet. According to her, her teacher had made it quite clear how the fingers must contact the strings. I did not arque with her.

"When you have your next lesson," I suggested, "ask your teacher about this."

When she came in for her next Alexander lesson she was smiling happily. "Judith," she said, "I showed Mr. Adams everything you showed me. He was very pleased. He said to me that two years ago he had tried to change the position of my shoulders and had given up in despair. He said also that the new fingering position is superior to the one I have been using!"

Bettina made rapid progress in her lessons, reinforcing and maintaining easy use of her body both in musical and everyday ways. She needed very few more lessons. Her playing improved and her body was free and dynamic. She was a different person.

When playing a musical instrument is a painful, cramped procedure, the music produced by such playing is also "cramped." When working with musicians, I have found that as they release, the tone of the instrument releases. As their ease and pleasure in the body becomes fuller, so does the music.

Violist Milton Thomas, who overcame a back problem through Alexander lessons, brought his viola to later lessons and played while I gave him directions. I angled these directions to maintain his good use while playing. He found, to his astonishment, that, expert as he was, his playing improved. His tone was more even.

"Judith, where did you learn to teach the viola?" he remarked one day. "You teach me the way I teach my students."

Some singers, dancers, musicians, and actors have a radiant or a magnetic air about them. There is a hush in the audience when they appear. And there is an undefinable stillness in the theater as they perform. Study such a person. He or she has good use of his or her body.

The late David Oistrakh, the famous Russian violinist, had admirable use of his body. The quality of his playing was as even and smooth as his ease of carriage.

Dietrich Fischer-Diskau (the famous tenor), Lord Laurence Olivier, Sir John Gielgud, Vivien Leigh, the late John Wayne, Margot Fonteyn, Mikhail Baryshnikov, all have a magnetism connected with remarkably good use of the body. Famous names, yes, but then the salesman who knows how to demonstrate a car without getting tense becomes just as successful in his field.

I remember Charles T., six feet three or four. As a sales representative, he drove his car many hours a day.

Charles was so tense, he could not smile. His shoulders were hunched up. He was apprehensive, nervous. At the first lesson he was fidgety about how he should sit or stand. It was hard to realize that inside that bundle of nerves there was even a teaspoonful of joy and well-being.

After two lessons, Charles began to smile. He was more at ease with me and with himself. Inside his tensed-up body, I began to see there really was a relaxed Charles trying to get out.

In two more lessons, he emerged, calm, poised, and joyous. "I still get tense though going from here to there," he said, meaning while driving and walking. He called both "work."

We discussed the thoughts he had. They were destination-oriented. He agreed to substitute Alexander directions as a replacement until his fixation of attention on "getting there" was non-existent.

I also spent a few minutes with him in the car. The construction of the seat is always of interest to me. If it is adverse to maintaining a lengthened back, then I recommend an adjustment in the seat or that a wedge be placed on the seat behind the back, the narrow edge of the wedge at the bottom, but *not* all the way down. Most auto supply firms carry this car seat wedge. They are inexpensive; in fact, the more expensive version in my experience, is not as good, as it has a hard wooden backing in it and is too rigid. What is needed is a support that is firm without being rigid. One may use a cushion instead of a wedge.

I also observe what students do with their legs while driving. Some people drive with their knees "stuck together." It is better to have knees apart. This promotes more ease in the legs, like the kind you experienced during the floor exercise, and release in the lower back and hip joints.

These are the kinds of recommendations I made for Charles. He cooperated and responded, reporting after a few more lessons, "I actually enjoy walking and driving." His work had turned to joy.

Misuse of the body becomes so "natural," once it becomes a habitual process, that we perpetuate it and reinforce it, totally unaware that we are doing so.

Good use of the body also becomes natural, and replaces misuse, once it has become habitual. Good use perpetuates and reinforces more good use.

I have used the term, "use of the body," as this is easier for you to understand. Actually, what we do with our bodies we are doing with *ourselves*, and Alexander's term *"use of the self"* is more accurate.

At my first Alexander lesson, my teacher, Judy Liebowitz, took polaroid photos of my front view and profile. When I saw them, I was horrified. I had had no idea I had such terrible posture.

"Who? Me? I never knew I looked so bad!" (See photos page 42.)

How about *you*, at this moment? Without moving, examine how you are sitting. It may feel comfortable to you, because it is *your* way of sitting, not someone else's way. Are your buttocks all the way back on the chair or couch? If not, you not only are interfering with a naturally lengthened back, but you are also forced to slump. The vertebrae are being squashed together, especially those in the lower back. This is one of the most common causes of lower back pain. It could also lead to sciatic pain in a leg. Some of you may *not* feel

SITTING ON A CHAIR

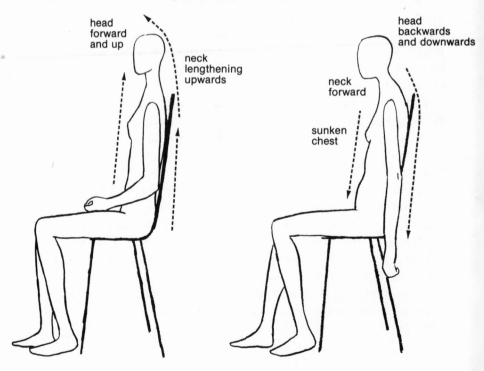

head
forward
and up

neck
lengthening
upwards

head
backwards
and downwards

neck
forward

sunken
chest

LENGTHENING   CONTRACTING

SITTING ON A CHAIR

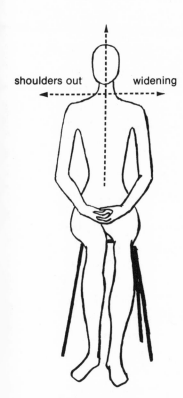

shoulders out   widening

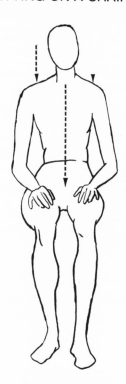

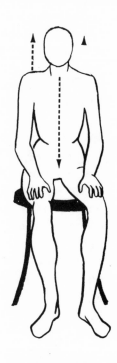

**LENGTHENING
AND WIDENING**

SLUMPED DOWN

**SLUMPED WITH
HUNCHED SHOULDERS**

SITTING ON THE FLOOR

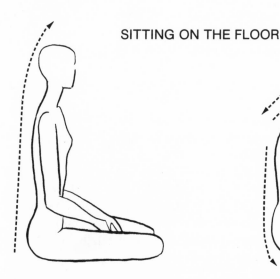

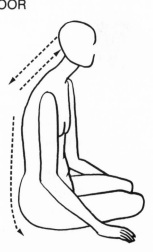

LENGTHENING UPWARDS

Note: chest and bosom uplift
and firm, toned abdomen

PULLED DOWN

Note: Sagging bosom
and protruding abdomen

comfortable with the way you are sitting now, and probably do not find *any* position comfortable. I used to be like that. What an unhappy way to go through life. With the Alexander Technique you can reverse this, so that you are *always* comfortable—and much happier with yourself.

▶ Habits That Wear Out Our Bodies

Don L., in his fifties, complained of an aching back and aching feet. He was a tall, slender, white-haired man.

More tall people are plagued by back pains than short people. I have no statistics on this, but I see this among my students and others. Perhaps it is because the center of gravity of tall people is high.

Don was an artist. Although his work was diversified, he was in demand to do portraits. Because of the painful aches he was experiencing standing at the easel, he had to accept fewer commissions to do these portraits, a lucrative part of his art. Usually there was a time element involved, and he sometimes could not meet the deadline because his painful back slowed him down. He had found a way of sitting on a chair to paint, but he said it was not satisfactory.

It was obvious in his first lessons that Don had developed some poor habits in standing and walking. He brought these poor habits to the easel where they were very harsh on his body because of the long hours he spent there.

If Don had not done something to improve his way of standing at the easel, the backaches would have quite likely led him to surgery, with attendant doubts and risks, in order to try and salvage his back and his career.

"Neck free, to let the head go forward and up, to let the back lengthen and widen" whispered mentally at the easel gave Don a new lease on his artistic life.

I have recommended that these thoughts be in your mind as you read this book. There are two purposes for this. First, if you are developing a bad reading habit—such as the body being held tense in some particular way—those words, conceptualized gently by you, can release some of the tension and partially or totally head off the development of a bad habit.

Second, by becoming familiar with the idea of the neck being free, and the head going forward and up, and the back lengthening and widening, you can play host to these ideas while going about your daily activities, and you may well be heading off other body habits that, through unnecessary tension, can cause wear and tear on muscle, bone, and inner organs. The benefit cannot be equivalent to the Alexander lesson where the teacher guides you directly in the "feeling" of good use, but it is a start. It is a start in a better direction and it may be just enough to ward off trouble.

Ernest was brought for Alexander lessons by his father. He was "eight going on nine." His father had had relief from a painful and numbing pinched nerve in the neck through Alexander lessons. Now he wanted help for his son because the boy was awkward in sports at school and was being jeered at by his fellow students.

He was a clumsy child, with a clownish walk. Little wonder Ernest was an unhappy boy. You could see it on his face and you could hear it in his barely audible voice.

We practically learned to walk all over again, Ernest and I. He forgot his physical body and thought of an imaginary one with a neck that was free, a head that went forward and up and a back that lengthened and widened, with the touch of my hands helping him experience this.

As his thoughts left his physical body, his movements became more harmonious. His walk normalized. His muscles were free to move in a coordinated way. He became less self-conscious as his body mimicked the image in his thought.

What good fortune that Ernest's father, instead of ridiculing him, led him to a more constructive way. His could have been the story of a boy who became an adult with many bad body habits, which is tantamount to a life sentence of poor health, pain, and unhappiness.

Instead, within a month Ernest was experiencing joy. You could see it on his face and you could hear it in his voice. His body moved gracefully, easily, smoothly. He would come running in to his lesson and tell me gleefully, "I run faster." "I got three hits yesterday," or "I made a double play."

A number of children have taken Alexander lessons because they were poor in gym or physical training and it was affecting their total school life. Youngsters are especially conscious of their body movement. They seek acceptance.

When this acceptance is threatened, it affects their whole outlook and sets the stage for poor mental, social and emotional habits.

If adults were as sensitive to their body misuse, they would be more motivated to identify and reverse these abuses.

An 8-year-old child was brought for Alexander lessons by her mother, as the mother was very unhappy with the awkwardness and poor posture of her young daughter. She had taken her daughter to other methods: ballet, postural exercises, gym, etc., and had found that instead of improving, the child was becoming worse.

These photos show the difference in the child after ten lessons in the Alexander Technique, taken once a week.

I had found this child extremely difficult to work with, as she was hyperactive; nonetheless, as evident in the pictures, there was a significant improvement. There was also an improvement in her behavior. By about the eighth lesson, she was less hyperactive.

➡ ## "It Is a Way of Life"

There are professionals who work with their hands, such as masseurs, chiropractors and physical therapists. There is a difference in the feel of the hands of, say, a masseuse after she has taken Alexander lessons.

Patients and clients of body therapists who have taken Alexander lessons report that there is a new quality in their work. This could merely be a by-product of a person's well-being—feel better and you do your work better. But there appears to be more to the phenomenon than this.

When a person who does body therapy has evolved a free body-mind partnership, it permits a purer flow of intuitive "knowing." The therapist's hands are automatically better able to do what needs to be done to the client when self-inhibiting factors have been removed.

One chiropractor told me, "I was giving myself Alexander directions while working on a patient with a long-standing back problem, who had been coming to me for a few months, and for the first time, I felt her spine release. She felt it, too."

When good direction for body use flows from the teacher to the student, the good direction in the student flows more easily; through this type of sequence, if the student is a therapist, it is then experienced by the patient as a healing touch.

Casual exposure to information about Alexander lessons can lead one to say, "Oh, that's for posture."

Yes, posture does improve, but that is a by-product. The Alexander Technique is *for life itself.* Gordon Davidson, Director of the Mark Taper Forum in Los Angeles, when asked once, "What is the Alexander Technique?" replied, *"It is a way of life."*

The old song about the knee bone being connected to the leg bone could be updated for the Technique.

The backbone is connected to the energy source.

The energy source is connected to creativity.

Creativity is connected to joy.

Joy is connected to love.

Love is connected to life.

➡ Tilting Knees to Release the Back

This gentle exercise can show you the connection between your legs, back, neck and head, and also the connection with your shoulder blades, shoulders and arms. By doing gentle movements with your knees you will feel a change in the other parts of your body.

This is a gentle, easy exercise that helps to unlock tension in the spine, in the back and in the neck, and result in more lengthening and widening. It is extremely simple to do, and is very pleasant and relaxing. It can also be fun.

Lie on a carpeted floor on your back, arms alongside your body and legs lying on the floor, spread apart comfortably.

Notice how your back is lying on the floor, and the back of your head. Notice the length of your legs, and how the backs of your legs feel as they lie on the floor? Notice your arms. Notice your breathing. Bring your attention to your lower belly and notice a very slight movement in your lower belly that is connected to your breathing. The muscles of your lower belly rise slightly up towards the ceiling and sink slightly down again.

Gently draw up your legs one at a time, so that your knees are bent

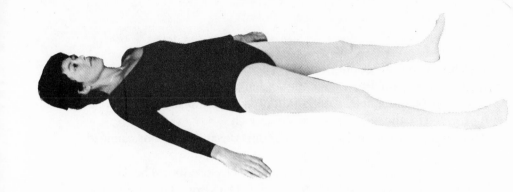

with your legs and feet spread apart. Spread your arms out at shoulder level, palms upwards. Slowly and gently tilt your knees right and left. Your head stays in the middle. See that your feet and legs remain spread apart, approximately the same width as the width across your shoulders. Notice the movement in your spine and your back, and how it travels all the way up to your head. Do this movement gently. As you continue doing the gentle movement with your knees, allow your head and eyes to roll right and left with the knees. Exhale each time you go to the side, and inhale as you pass through the middle. It is even more helpful to exhale through your mouth. Open your mouth to exhale, and close it as you inhale. Do medium-size movements, not big and not small.

Now come to the middle and leave your head in the middle. Lower your legs to the floor gently one at a time, and lie on the floor with your legs spread apart, arms alongside you and again sense your body. See how your back is lying on the floor, and your legs, your arms, and your head. Are there any changes in the way you are lying on the floor?

After you have rested, draw up your legs one at a time and bring your legs into the same position that they were in before. Spread your arms out at shoulder level with your palms upward. Tilt your knees right and left, and let your head and eyes roll gently in the opposite direction to your knees. This corkscrew movement of the spine has a marvelous effect on your neck and back. Have you started to hold your breath? Allow your breath to softly flow out of your mouth as you turn your head to the side, and inhale as you pass through the middle. Gently swing your knees right and left, right and left, and let your head and eyes roll opposite to the knees. What a pleasurable feeling it can be to move your spine and your back in a way that can undo knots and tensions and erase stress.

Let this become a little faster, more playful. Do not hold your breath, and do not rush. Have fun with it. After you have done it this way for a while, let your head and eyes roll in the same direction as your knees, from side to side.

Now stay in the middle and slowly lower your arms and your legs and close your eyes and rest here. Be aware of changes in yourself.

After a while, slowly come to standing by drawing up your knees and rolling to one side onto your hands and knees and then up to standing. Do you feel different as you come up to standing, and walk around the room? Are you walking like a different person? Do you feel that stress has been wiped out of your back and your neck? As you walk, turn your head gently from side to side. Does your neck feel easier? Look at yourself in a mirror. Are your eyes more shiny, your skin more glowing? Is your torso more erect, are your shoulders broader?

These are simple gentle movements that can bring more life to you, rejuvenate you, open you up to more feeling, more joy. These are movements that are kind to you, and good to you, and also can be fun.

➡ Beyond Good Posture

People often go through an entire lifetime being a slave to their bodies. From the hypochondriac to the "health nut," there are those who do not freely use their bodies but are imprisoned by them.

For some people, survival is a battle against the intimidations of the body. They need pills to sleep, pills to quiet their nerves, pills to stop headaches. And then they take pills to help alleviate the effects on the body of the other pills.

For them, body liberation means liberation from the body—the kind that comes with death.

It does not have to be this way.

Many of those who come for Alexander lessons are daily relying on pain-relieving pills. Through the improved use of their bodies, they get relief from pain and release from the pills. The Technique does not, as far as I know, eliminate ailments such as calcium deposits, damaged vertebrae, slipped discs; nor does it bring back to life dead muscles such as those in a victim of polio.

How does relief from pain come about? It is difficult to know exactly what happens. What I see is that with the lightening and lengthening comes a release of downward pressure in the body, and with it relief from pressure on the vulnerable area. It is primarily muscular pressure, but this in turn pulls down the various parts of the skeleton, as well as squashing down on various internal organs. It could also be applying pressure to veins and capillaries. Release the pressure and you may relieve the pain.

Sometimes there is no damage in any part of the body, according to the physician, and yet the person is in pain; this is often the case with back pain. I would say that in these instances the problem is muscular tension, or what we call "contraction."

One of my students was a man on heavy medication because of severe chest pains. He was referred to me by his psychiatrist, whom he had been seeing for several years. The psychiatrist told me later that he was treating this patient for anxiety.

The man was "hyperactive." He walked fast, talked fast, could not be still, in short, came across as a bundle of nerves. He was short and stocky, and I immediately observed a great deal of tension in his body, especially severe in the neck, chest and legs. He had a heavy, jerky walk, and walked slightly sideways; his eyes never looked straight ahead, always moving from one side to the other. He did not smile.

He told me he had suffered from chest pains for a few years. As they had become worse, he had increased his daily medication. The chest pains felt to him as if he were having a heart attack. Even while he was on the medication, he would sometimes suddenly get a severe attack of pain, would be rushed to the emergency room of the hospital, would be tested for heart trouble, and was always told there was nothing wrong with his heart. And he was given more medi- cation.

This man had had no exposure to any body methods, or mind- body awareness techniques, and could not understand how the Technique might be helpful. The work seemed insignificant to him, and he continued the lessons only because his psychiatrist had prescribed them for him.

He drove a long way after work, two to three times a week, for the lessons. After one week he was starting to feel improvement but said he did not see how it could be connected to the Alexander work. He had no idea what might have brought about the improvement. He explained that he had been living with the feeling of severe tension in his chest and the fear that another "attack" might occur at any moment. He had one attack since he started lessons, but it had not lasted long and had been less severe. He was now sensing less tension in his chest. Soon after, he was mostly free of tension and the ensuing anxiety, it occurred only when he drove to and from work; later it occurred only when driving to work and eventually not at all. He went through a period of expecting it to return, and finally that anxiety dissipated itself. He had gradually reduced his medication to nil, and was taking lessons only once a week. By this time he was convinced that the change was a result of the lessons, and his psychiatrist concurred.

The man was now cheerful, relaxed, free of pain, tension and anxiety. He had developed a reputation for being the most relaxed person at work. It was less than two months since his first Alexander lesson. He cheerfully discontinued his lessons, feeling confidence in his newfound self.

➡ The Power of Choice

We all have the power to choose. Many of us do not realize this, as we go through life doing everything the same way as we have always done it. In many situations, if we would stop for a split second we would give ourselves a chance to realize that there is more than one way to do things.

In the Alexander Technique, we apply this to the movements of our everyday life. For example, when you want to sit down, take a split second to stop, so that you can "inhibit" your usual poor habits, and you have a chance to move well—*you have the choice* to go to the chair with poor use or with good use.

We all have natural, good use within us, and we interfere with it with our poor habitual responses. You can put a stop to that by stopping for a split second. In that split second, you can give your

Alexander directions, and allow your movement to happen easily as you continue to think of your head going forward and up and your back lengthening.

You can use this "split second to stop" just before *any* movement. In the middle of a movement it would usually be unnatural to stop. However, you could *think of stopping* and give your directions *without actually stopping*. The most important time to stop, is just before you start to do something, and I think you will find as a result that you move with more ease and flow.

When you apply this principle of "knowing how to stop" to other areas of your life, it can help you change other unwanted habits. Let us take overeating as an example. As soon as you feel that you want to reach for a cookie, stop for a split second, say no to doing your usual activity; in that split second you have allowed yourself other alternatives, other choices. *When you know how to stop, you give yourself choice.* You can choose to do something else. With this power of choice, you might choose to go for the cookie, then you do it through conscious choice, rather than mindless compulsion. At another time, you might choose not to go for the cookie, and choose to do something else, perhaps turn on the radio to some lively music and dance to it or take care of something that needs to be taken care of. Instead of eating the cookie, you might choose to do something constructive, and it may be something that is fun. We could call this "constructive thinking." Use constructive thinking to help your relations with other people, those you work with and friends and lovers. When you are about to say something out of resentment because you are angry, or feel hurt, take that split second to stop. You give yourself the choice to say something else if you want to. Perhaps you will choose to say the very thing you intended to, and you go ahead and do so. It is a different experience when you do it through choice. The power of reasoned choice differentiates us from animals. This is what makes you a human being, and especially an adult, mature human being. Through this, you can make your life freer and happier, free from compulsion, and more joyous.

◗ The Psychophysical Experience

The body is a beautiful mechanism designed to serve us. It works beautifully for people who know how to care for it and use it well. Unfortunately, those who do not know are permitting them-selves to be the slaves of their own servo-mechanism.

"Knowing" means proper use. Used properly, the body performs the master's bidding. If that bidding is sleep, sleep comes. If that bidding is a call for energy, there is energy to spare. If that bidding is to perform a particular skill, the skillfulness appears without sweat and tears.

I have sometimes conveyed to my students that the mind is like the master of a household. The master stands at the head of the staircase and gives orders to the servants. The servants carry out the orders efficiently, and the master does not go down among them and carry out the work.

In Alexander, the orders are the mental directions. The body parts are the servants who carry out the master's orders, and they know how to do it. The mind—the master—*only gives the orders* and is not involved with even thinking of doing the activity. He *directs* the whole procedure.

One day, to my surprise, I read the same concept in a translation of ancient documents on the Chinese art of T'ai chi.

Body and mind work as a team. When each knows its role, and does not interfere with the role of the other, there is a harmonious interrelationship that allows greater fulfillment. This is the *body-mind* relationship, or, in other words, the *psychophysical* ex-perience.

Dancers, particularly ballet dancers, who have become aware of the difference between good use and poor use and who have rein-stated their good use through Alexander lessons, report a new ease and joy in their dancing, replacing hard work and strain.

"I always thought dancing had to be hard work at the bar, and strain before an audience," said one. "My ballet teacher had always told me if it doesn't hurt it's no good. I have discovered that Alexan-der directions make pain and strain obsolete. I can now achieve more with my body at the exercise bar, with ease, and perform better before an audience. Instead of sweat and torture, I feel exhilaration and joy." Others echo her. "This is what dancing ought to feel like!"

Ballet dancers find that their legs fly higher, their pirouettes are faster, their balance is better and their movements are smoother—

all with less practice at the bar. It is as if the body no longer opposes, but cooperates. The mechanism of the body serves well, and there is an indescribable improvement in quality.

When a body is free of the "programmings" from the stresses of the world around it, it is able to respond more exquisitely to demands for movement, skill, artistry and creativity.

"I leap higher." "I balance better." "I learn difficult movements more easily."

Can you say that this is all due to better posture? It is due to better direction. The mind, burdened with anxiety and stress, gives faulty directions. When those directions are eliminated, joy enters.

▶ Raising Arms and Legs With Direction

There are many times in your daily life when you need to reach up for something, and most of us over-work while doing it. Perhaps I can help you experience the difference between good use and poor use through these simple movements of raising the arms, and also moving the legs.

Stand comfortably facing a mirror, so that you can see your upper torso. You will feel the effect without a mirror, and with a mirror you may actually see some change in your body.

Stand with your feet comfortably apart. Raise your right arm as if you are reaching for something, and reach up as high as you can with your arm, without going on your toes, stretching your right arm upwards. I think you will find that it is quite an effort, in your shoulder and neck as well as in your arm. Lower your arm and swing it softly forwards and backwards to gently shake out some of the tension that came into your arm from stretching upwards strenuously. Now let your arm rest.

I will now ask you to do the same movement with your Alexander directions, and I will also give you an additional helpful thought. Before you do anything about raising your arm, I would like you to allow your chin to lower slightly and tell your head it is going forward and up and think of your torso lengthening upwards, following your head. Imagine that your head cannot go up without your torso also lengthening upwards. While you remind yourself of your head going forward and up and your back lengthening upwards, allow your right arm to float up in the air *and think of the fingertips of your right hand leading the movement of your arm*. At the same time, your head is leading the movement of your torso upwards. *It is pure thought*. You allow your fingertips and arm to float upwards. Please do *not* stretch your arm upwards, *let it float up*. When it is up in the air, think of your fingertips floating further up, and your arm lengthening and allow your fingertips to move a little further, as if it is your fingertips that are reaching for something; at the same time, tell your head it is continuing to go forward and up, and your back is continuing to lengthen.

To bring your arm down, tell your head to go forward and up and your back to lengthen, and *allow your fingertips to float gently downwards*. Naturally when your fingertips float down, your arm also floats down. Now you have *counter-direction*: while your fingertips and arm float downwards, your head and torso are directed upwards. When your arm has come down think of your length again. Repeat this experience with your right arm one or two times.

Now stand with your arms hanging easily at your sides, and see whether your right arm feels longer and lighter, and perhaps the right side of your torso, including the right side of your neck, feels lighter and longer. Look in the mirror, and perhaps you can see that the right side of your body is longer and that your right arm is now longer than the left. Think of how that movement felt when you did it with Alexander direction, as compared to how you did it earlier, forcing it to stretch upward. Didn't it feel easier when you did it gently and softly with your thoughts guiding your muscles? You can make all your movements easier by using your thoughts to direct them. Walk around and see if you feel a difference between your right side and your left side.

Do this now on the left side. After having done it on your left side, you are likely to feel that your whole torso is lighter, and that the two sides are equally light and long as well as both arms feeling equally light and long. Perhaps your head is lighter, resting more lightly on the top of your spine; does it feel that it is going upwards towards the ceiling, rather than settling down onto your neck?

In this "Alexander experience," I added the thought of letting your fingertips lead the movement of your arm. When you use the idea of your *fingertips leading*, instead of thinking of moving your arm, the arm moves more easily and the movement in the shoulder joint is freer. This is a very helpful idea that you can use for your other limbs also. It is particularly useful for dancers and for exercises.

When you are actually reaching up for an object, the movement is a little different, although the mental directions are the same. As you can see in the figures below, reaching up for something involves going up on the toes and also looking up at the object. You still direct "neck free, head forward and up, back lengthening and widening," and you direct yourself in this way before going up onto your toes and before you raise your arm and before you look up; you direct yourself again while you go onto your toes, raise your arms, and look upwards. However, you could use two additional thoughts while doing

REACHING UPWARDS

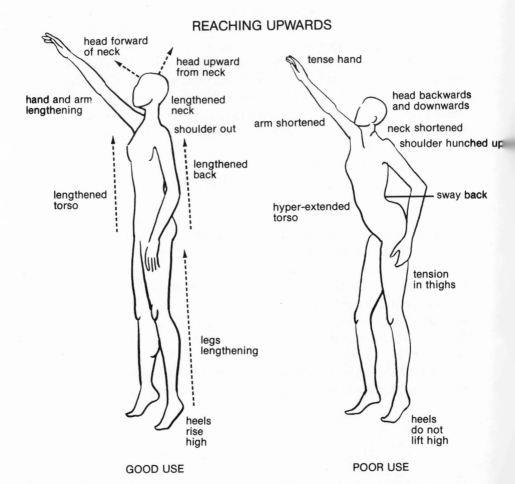

head forward of neck

head upward from neck

tense hand

hand and arm lengthening

lengthened neck

head backwards and downwards

shoulder out

arm shortened

neck shortened

shoulder hunched up

lengthened back

lengthened torso

sway back

hyper-extended torso

tension in thighs

legs lengthening

heels rise high

heels do not lift high

GOOD USE

POOR USE

these actions: you *look upwards with length*, and *your fingertips float upwards* towards the object. As you bring the object down, you again direct neck free, head forward and up, back lengthening and widening, and you add the thought that *your fingertips are floating downwards*. When you have brought the object down, you again direct your neck, head and back. Whatever your activity, it is best to direct *before, during and after*, and to *think of everything you do as the act of lengthening*.

Notice that with poor use the whole body contracts and shortens, and therefore is not as functional: you cannot reach as far as with good use. These drawings were drawn from a live model demonstrating the difference between good use and poor use and are therefore quite accurate in demonstrating the differences.

I would like to show how dancers can improve their movements; dancers do more exaggerated movements than we do in daily life, and an idea can be shown more clearly in an exaggerated movement. Dancers frequently raise their arms; sometimes they raise them with elbows straight and the fingers dangling down; sometimes they riase them with the arms straight and hands straight, fingers pointing ahead; sometimes they raise an arm with the elbow bent. For each one of these movements, I would give a different thought. The thoughts I am going to suggest are most effective when given *in addition* to thoughts of your head going forward and up and your back lengthening. Please do not use them as a substitute; they will not have as much benefit as when you add them to your basic Alexander thoughts. At this stage you may not need to say all the words of the Alexander thoughts and can use one thought, for example, "lengthening," or "head going up."

I will talk of a dancer raising one arm, as it will be easier to explain, however, what I say applies also to raising both arms. When raising an arm with the elbow straight and the wrist straight, hands and fingers pointing ahead, I suggest thinking of the fingertips leading, then the whole arm moves upwards with ease and grace. When the arm comes down, think of the fingertips floating downwards, while the head and back are going upwards.

Let us take another movement of the arm going up. This time the elbow is straight, and the hand is dangling down from the wrist. In this instance, it is the wrist that is leading the arm upwards, and I would suggest thinking of the wrist floating up. However, on the way down, when the hand is dangling down, the fingertips would be leading the downward movement, and I would suggest thinking of the fingertips floating down.

Another movement is raising the arm with the elbow bent, and the elbow is leading the arm upwards. I would suggest thinking of the elbow floating upwards, and for coming down think of the elbow floating downwards, all the while directing head and back to go upwards.

We can apply the same ideas to the legs. In the movement of raising the leg with a pointed toe, the toes are leading. Think of the toes floating upwards and the leg lengthening, and on the way down, think of the toes floating downwards. In some movements, the leg is raised with a bend at the ankle, and the toes are pointing upwards. In this movement it is the heel that is leading, and you would think of your heel floating upwards, and the leg lengthening. When lowering the leg, think of your heel floating downwards and the leg lengthening. You may actually feel your leg getting longer, lighter, and more graceful.

Another way to raise the leg is by bending the knee. Now the knee is leading the movement, and you need to think of your knee floating upwards and your knee floating downwards. I would like to remind you that all these thoughts of toes, elbows, wrists, fingers, heel or knee leading, are to be given *in addition to Alexander neck-head-back directions*.

These ideas are excellent for many activities, including some of the ordinary movements of daily life. Other activities where you can use them are in sports, athletics, gymnastics, and any other area that you can think of.

I have found these ideas very helpful for people who have had an injury in a limb, or have had surgery, such as knee surgery, and are having difficulty moving the limb.

Instead of thinking of the whole leg or the whole arm moving, think of the part that is leading the movement and direct that part to float upwards or float downwards, and your arm or leg will move far more easily.

You can apply these thoughts when you are doing movements with your legs or arms in any position, while sitting or while lying down, they are not confined exclusively to standing up.

➡ Getting Out of Our Own Way

A German professor, Eugen Herrigel, wrote a book entitled *Zen in the Art of Archery*, about his study of archery in Japan under a Zen master. Herrigel's master sounds very much like F.M. Alexander in his approach to the mind-body relationship.

The master exhorted his pupils to get out of their own way, to not become emotionally involved with reaching the target; or with the act of letting the arrow fly, and to let the bow do it. Herrigel had to learn to draw the bow yet not draw it, to allow the arrow to remove itself from his hand and take flight toward the target of its own accord. Years later, when he had finally mastered this art of not getting in his own way, he was not permitted to become elated over it. He had not really done something right, he had merely *stopped doing many things wrong.*

When we stop doing things wrong, we are on the path to fulfillment.

Chapter 7

How to Give Yourself Directions: Lying, Sitting, Standing and Walking

THE SWITCH FROM ONE PATH to another begins here and now. It need not wait until trouble rears its painful head. You can begin to sit, stand, lie, and walk in ways which are free of stress and humanly natural. By beginning with these fundamental body uses, other uses fall naturally into the same free and harmonious pattern. The catalyst behind this switch is mental direction.

When you give yourself mental direction, you can feel as if you have taken off tight-fitting foundation garments or have come out of a restricting, ill-fitting suit.

Just as the ballet dancer reports an improvement in every aspect of dancing, you can feel a new freedom in your "dance" through life. Every movement benefits. Going from here to there, working at a desk, driving, exercising, playing at a sport—all become free and easy as if you had lost ballast that had been holding you down. You have seen pictures of space walkers and noticed the ease with which they glide from here to there; that is the kind of lightness that body movement seems to take on.

You can zero in on a particular movement and by giving the Alexander directions to yourself while doing this movement you will transform what is the hard work of your day into no work that is effortless.

A Laughing Matter

Norman Cousins, former editor of *Saturday Review*, was taken seriously ill some years ago. A paralysis was rapidly worsening. His doctor had diagnosed it as collagen breakdown. The condition did not respond to treatment and his doctor began to consider the illness as terminal.

Cousins decided that he must take charge if he was to survive.

Acting as his own doctor, he prescribed for himself massive doses of vitamin C and shortly after added a prescription for laughter. He watched old Marx Brothers movies and reel after reel of "Candid Camera." By the eighth day of this treatment, the progression of the paralysis had stopped and begun to reverse.

Cousins has told his story in his book *Anatomy of an Illness as Perceived by the Patient*.

Laughter is good medicine. Laughter is an antidote for killer stress. Stress kills slowly, little by little, wearing us down and wearing us out. Laughter can reverse the process. It is a good way to release tensions throughout the body in addition to the restorative and corrective mental directions. With a good spell of laughter, the muscles of your body relax as though you had taken a warm bath. You have washed away the grime of stress and are ready for the glow and reflection of easier body use.

➡ Getting To Know Your Body Better

In a moment we are going to laugh. But first, let us get to know our body better. Stand up, your feet comfortably apart.

How do you feel standing here? Notice the back of your neck. Notice how your lower back feels. Travel up your back and become aware of how your upper back and shoulder blades feel. How does your head feel on top of your spine? Does it feel as if it is poised lightly or does it feel like a heavy weight? Be aware of your arms. How do they feel? Heavy? Light? Weightless or weighty? How do your legs feel? Tense? Loose? In-between?

What is your mind doing? What is it thinking about?

If you like, make written notes about what you have come up with. List the feelings that you have detected, good or bad, and the thoughts you were having.

Now let's laugh. Let's laugh right now. Laugh out loud. If you are embarrassed to laugh because there are other people in the room or within hearing distance, find a private, insulated spot like the bathroom or a closet or your car, where you can be alone and rock with laughter. Or, you can invite others to join you.

You can buy a laughing record that is quite infectious, or you can wait for some slapstick comedy on television, or you can picture things in your mind that will make you laugh.

Resist the tendency to tell yourself, "I know what it feels like to laugh, let's get on with it." If you feel that tendency, you may need the warm bath of laughter more than some others.

Can you see somebody you dislike getting a pie thrown in his face?

Can you see a fat man wobbling on ice skates?

Laugh!

Let the laughter roll and rollick from you!

Stand up and laugh.

Notice what your body does while you are laughing. Do you throw your head back? How does the back of your neck feel? Which muscles shake you?

Some of our habits reveal themselves while laughing. Observe your mannerisms as you laugh. A person who brings his shoulders up to his ears while laughing is likely to be tensing his shoulders in this way in other situations. Did you sway your back or tense your neck while laughing? This may indicate a propensity to do this in other activities. What we do in one activity tends to be a constant habit that appears in other activities, sometimes more so, sometimes less so. Did your knees buckle? Did your knees lock? Locked knees are indicative of rigidity in a person. Buckling knees are an indication of a soft or wishy-washy person.

The body habits I just described can interfere with joy and exhilaration. It happens in laughing just as it does in other activities of life.

Those who laugh freely sense a joyousness which continues after they stop laughing. The face is rosy and the eyes glowing. A feeling of exhilaration after a good laugh indicates a quickening of the blood supply to reach through tiny capillaries to the cells of the body and brain that might be starved for oxygen.

Remove the repressive habits, substitute, through good direction, a more normal use of the body, and joy is no longer inhibited, no longer bottled up by habits that are like the shadow of rigor mortis on its way.

Now stand, feet comfortably apart, arms by your sides, and go over the feeling of your body the way you did before the laughing spell. Again be aware of the subtle feelings of neck, head, back, arms and legs, and what your thoughts are doing.

Write these impressions down on another sheet of paper. Now compare what you just wrote to what you wrote before. Notice the differences. Allow the changes to enhance your perception of your body.

Your body is in constant change.

The cells in your body are replaced within a year. New cells will grow either in a climate of mental serenity or of mental stress. It makes a difference to those cells. As periods of serenity or stress come and go, the body reacts to them, just as your body reacted to the period of laughter you just experienced.

Alexander directions allow a climate of serenity, mental and physical.

➡ Alexander Directions: The Effect On You

The idea of your neck being free is a novel one.

You did not learn about freeing your neck in school, in family life, or in your job.

The idea of your head going forward and up is also a novel one. Whoever has talked to you of that kind of a concept before? And what about the back lengthening and widening? Who would ever propose that to you?

You have heard these three concepts over and over in this book. As you sit here reading now, you may already feel somewhat different than you did when you started Chapter I. By reading about these directions again and again, and automatically conceptualizing them, you have been reacting to them. The difference you feel may be subtle or it may be obvious. The difference is the road toward freedom and fluidity.

This difference is now going to be increased. In this chapter, we are going to go further in discussing these directions and applying them to more movements. This means that your concepts of your neck, head and back will become more focused and will have even more effect on your body, an effect that can begin to release you from your unwanted past and introduce you to new levels of present joy and satisfaction.

"My body feels lighter."

"I am sitting more erect."

These are statements of people who merely hear or read about the Alexander Technique. There is no way to read and not conceptualize. If I were to mention a white polar bear in a pink bikini, there is no way for your mind to escape the concept. Maybe this concept will be fuzzy, it may not be in vivid technicolor, but it is there. Once the concept of your head going forward and up is there, there is no way for you to avoid a response.

▶ Table Work—Or Lying Down

Alexander directions often have very clear effects in table work. The student lies on the table, with books under the head, as neck, head and back instructions are given, together with the teacher's gentle touch. The directions are the same, except that "head forward and up" becomes "head forward and *out*." Many students experience the table work as blissful and delicious.

On the table, the student does nothing except lie there, with eyes open. The teacher goes to the head, neck, spine, legs, shoulders and arms giving the directions. The knees of the student are moved up by the teacher to a bent position, and occasionally brought down and up again; shoulders are smoothed out by the teacher, and the back encouraged to elongate; all this is done to the "tune" of the Alexander directions.

It is initially easier for the student to experience the Alexander directions while lying down, being supported by the table. The muscles of the back and neck do not have to work while prone, and

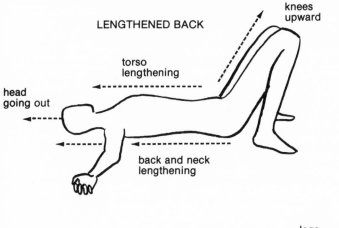

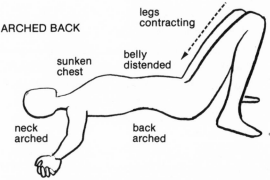

they are able to respond more easily to the directions. The lengthening is usually quite extensive and I have to move the head support backwards several times to accommodate the lengthening back.

Table work is valuable as the student is not involved in any other activity, and can easily experience lengthening. Also, lying down is one of our regular activities. Many of us lie down with a tight, arched lower back—a mouse could run through the space under the back. Consequently, shoulders, arms, and legs are tight, to say nothing of the neck. On the table, the back flattens, the shoulders broaden, and legs elongate while the teacher and student direct length and the teacher uses his or her hands with Alexandrian expertise.

The experience is the fundamental teacher. Direct. Lengthen. Direct. Lengthen. All this happens quite fast on the table.

One of my students, a 60-year-old woman, told me one day that she had been thrown off her horse, and had landed flat on her back *without hurting herself.* She said, "I fell with softness." I like to think that the table work had helped her.

While on the table, the student may add additional directions, such as "knees up" which directs the knees upward toward the ceiling; and "shoulders out" which directs the left shoulder to the left wall and the right shoulder toward the right wall. These directions are to be said quickly and lightly, in *addition* to the basic directions, and are *not* to replace them. Here is a suggestion for directing on the table: "Neck free, head forward and out, back lengthening and widening, knees up, shoulders out, neck free, head forward and out. . . ."

Table work is invaluable for those who cannot sit. I have worked with people who have muscular sclerosis who could not sit or stand, and they have had very gratifying improvements with table work.

Some back problems are so severely painful that the person cannot sit or stand. In some of these cases, the physician has ordered complete bed rest for several weeks. The same has applied to those who had just had back surgery. After a few table lessons, these people have been able to sit, walk and stand sufficiently to have "chair work," and it has not taken long before they have been functioning normally again.

Those with a delicate spine, or spinal problem, need a little extra padding under the lower back while lying on the table. A soft pillow helps, but in severe cases even that applies painful pressure. The answer is a "doughnut."

A doughnut is an inflatable rubber cushion that has a hole in the center, just like a doughnut.

Most drugstores stock this item. If unavailable, one can make something similar with foam rubber. It is round, slightly smaller

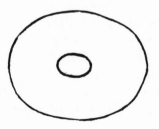
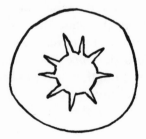

than a toilet seat, with a smaller hole than a toilet seat, the hole being approximately 4–5 inches in diameter. It should not be very thick. When using foam rubber, you would need to make a few slashes around the hole, to soften the surrounding area.

The delicate part of the spine lies over the hole and in this way nothing is in contact with it to hurt it.

Those of you whose lower back aches when lying down could benefit from placing a doughnut under your lower back. And remember to bend your knees when lying down. With Alexander lessons, the doughnut after a while has usually become unnecessary.

Most, but not all Alexander teachers include table work in their lessons. Among them, some prefer to do it at the beginning of the lesson, and some at the end.

I like to vary. With beginning students my preference is to start with table work, as it is easier on both student and teacher; the student comes up off the table with a head start. This means a lighter, easier, more malleable body, as well as visible improvement in the alignment. The chair work is easier with a body that has already been "directed."

Most of the students are eager to lie on the table and be "Alexandered." Their only activity is to "direct" themselves, through the Alexander thoughts, and this to them is an introduction to *nondoing*. They yield to the teacher's hands and to the delicious sensations of lengthening, flattening out along the table, and becoming smoother, as they allow contraction to ease out of the body.

One woman loved this so much, she said to me one day, "Judith, this is such bliss. Will you marry me?"

You can direct yourself without a teacher while lying down. Lie on the floor or on a table, or on some other flat surface with some padding so that your spine is not lying on a hard surface. Carpeting on the floor or a foam pad on the table will do. Or, use blankets or a sleeping bag. It is important that there be some cushioning for your spine.

Put one, two or three paperback books under your head. Use enough to make your head comfortable. In some cities the telephone directory is the ideal height. Leave your eyes open, blinking normally.

Bend first one knee, then the other, and spread your legs and feet comfortably apart. Now your are in the position that is most advantageous for lengthening while lying down.

How would you give the basic Alexander directions, "Let the neck be free, to let the head go forward and out, to let the back lengthen and widen." Would you do it? Say it? Think it?

The first thing to remember is to not *do* anything. Do not even close your eyes. The next thing to remember is to not *say* anything aloud. *Think* comes closest to it. You could visualize. Or you could say the words *silently*, as if giving a command.

➡ Images Versus Commands

Although not all Alexander teachers may agree on this, visualization, in my experience, is not as effective as thinking of the words as *specific orders* to be obeyed.

I often use mental images to help my students capture the concept required, but I ask them not to rely on visualization, or images. I discourage *continuous use* of visualization or mental picturing by my students for two reasons:

1. The effect does not last over a long period of time.
2. It takes longer to visualize a picture than to say a brief command.

I discovered from my students early in my teaching practice that an image used repeatedly loses its "strength." It is no longer effective in Alexander work after repeated use. You can argue that the same is true of words, that, when said over and over again, words lose their initial impact. The words, however, develop an association through the effect of the Alexander teacher's hands. The words define and reinforce that experience. Perhaps this is because words are the medium of communication between teacher and student.

After a brief period of lessons, a triggering action is caused by simply saying mentally the first word, "Let," or "Neck." The whole sequence is initiated by thinking this. The word is faster than visualizing an image Even when you are using the three complete phrases of the directions, you can say them quite fast. Thinking them silently is much more rapid than saying words aloud. Try it for yourself and compare.

Most people require more time than that to conjure up an image. First they have to decide *which image* to use, then proceed to bring all the various parts of the image into place. At the beginning of this book I asked you to think of your head being a balloon floating upwards and curving gently forward at the same time, as if wafted by a breeze. See how much time it takes to put into place all the pieces of the picture: yourself, your head, the balloon, the breeze. Now silently say "Head forward and up" quickly and see how much time that takes.

I find that often *images are invaluable and irreplaceable for an initial understanding*: they are enlightening. Once you have understood the concept with the help of an image and experienced the effect, then you can connect the experience with the words, and from then on the words will do the job every time. It will also work using different words, if you wish.

The Alexander Technique is for your daily life. How cumbersome it would be for you to have to interrupt activities, either alone or with other people, to conjure up pictures. This cumbersomeness actually interferes with the easy flow of good use. Instead, a word or two said rapidly and silently can be easily interjected at any time. Saying the words can become a reflex action that is as fast as hitting the brake with your foot when you see a red light. And the response in your body to the words is just as instantaneous.

You will note that the teacher is a factor in enhancing the connection between words and feeling, and since the light touch of an Alexander teacher is not providing part of the experience for you, it may be that the words will not hold as great an advantage over the image when learning via this book. However, I still recommend that you direct in your daily life by giving mental "orders," because speed is important. Joy belongs in your daily life. The more time it takes to turn it on, the less you will avail yourself of it. The less time it takes, the more you will avail yourself of it.

I could give you all kinds of visual suggestions—picturing a string pulling your head forward and up; seeing yourself as a tree with the sap flowing up the trunk and out into the branches—but your own commands, mentally verbalized, are faster and more effective on a daily basis.

When an Alexander student, who has had a few lessons, is bending down to open a drawer and feels tension, all that student needs to do is mentally think the command "lengthen" or "neck free" and the whole body releases its tension instantly. It is a learned or "conditioned" response, due to the words and touch of the teacher.

You, the reader, are without the experience of a teacher, and yet I recommend the mental words as the means to give yourself good direction.

Use images for your initial learning, to help bring about the first experiences.

Use mental commands on a daily basis.

➡ A Mini-Alexander Lesson or Self-Alexandering

I would like to guide you in giving yourself a mini-Alexander lesson while lying down, using a combination of visual images and Alexander mental directions.

Lie down on the floor, with enough cushioning or carpeting under your back for you to be comfortable, and the required number of paperbacks under your head to allow your head and neck to lengthen outwards. Lie with your legs resting on the floor, feet spread fairly wide apart, approximately the same width as the width of your shoulders.

As you do not have an Alexander teacher with you to bend your legs for you, I would like to show you a way to do it for yourself, and perhaps you will get some of the same experience as you would get with an Alexander teacher.

First of all, let us see what it is like to bend your knees without Alexander direction. While you lie here, simply bend one knee, and then bend the other knee, so that you are lying on the floor with both knees bent and soles of both feet placed on the floor. Now lower one leg to the floor, and then lower the other leg. Let your legs and feet be fairly wide apart, as before. Do it once more, and as you do it notice how your legs feel and how your back feels. Leave your legs lying on the floor.

Let us do it now in an Alexandrian way. I am going to give you an additional thought.

I will ask you to give your mental directions, lightly, easily and casually. Tell your head to go out behind you, and you could pretend that there is no wall there, and your head goes out to infinity. Let us pretend that your spine and back are made of elastic, and that the lower part of your spine, the tail bone, is lightly glued to the floor. While your head goes out your back and spine are lengthening because they are attached to the head. They get longer and longer, and longer. Your head is leading the length. As you give yourself these thoughts lightly and easily, think of your right knee; pretend that there is a string attached to your right knee, which is going up towards the ceiling, and that someone is holding the string in his hands. Again, think of your head going out and your back lengthening, and think that this invisible person is lifting the string up towards the ceiling, as if he is a puppeteer and your knee is a puppet. As he lifts the string towards the ceiling, your knee starts to move up towards the ceiling. Allow your knee to bend following your thought of the puppeteer moving the string upwards. Also think of your head going out and your back lengthening. Finally your knee is fully bent and the sole of your right foot is resting on the floor. Place your foot down somewhat to the right of center, not close to the center.

Think again of your head going out and your back lengthening, and now think of your left knee, and imagine the puppeteer holding up a string attached to your left knee. While you tell your head to go out and your back to lengthen, you allow your knee to move upwards, as if the puppeteer is pulling the string up and bending your knee for you. Finally your left foot is resting on the floor, and your knee is bent.

It is important that you do these movements slowly, so that you have time to direct with your mind. It does not need to be at a snail's pace, which is laborious, but do not rush through these movements.

Repeat this experience, doing it at a pace that is soft and gentle. As you do it, see whether your knees and your legs feel different, and whether your back feels different when you do it with your imaginary puppeteer moving your knees upwards, while your head is going out and your back lengthening. Is this a different experience than your first one, when you thought of nothing but the act of getting your knees up? When you arrive with your knees bent and the soles of your feet resting on the floor, does your back feel different against the floor? What about your neck and your head, your shoulder blades and your arms?

Let us explore an easy way to bring the legs down. Tell your head it is going out, tell your back it is lengthening, breathe normally and blink normally, so that the mental directions do not interfere with your normal functions. As you give yourself the thoughts, allow your left heel to slowly and gently slide down the floor, until it cannot slide any further and your left leg is lying on the floor. How did that feel compared to the way you first brought your leg down?

Again, think of your head going out and your back lengthening, and think of your right heel. You can pretend that there is a string attached to your right heel, and an invisible puppeteer starts to pull that string so that your right heel glides down the floor, and all the time you are directing your head to go out in the opposite direction than the heel. You have *counter-direction*: the heel and leg going in one direction, and the head and torso in the other direction. Your heel softly and gently slides down the floor, until your leg is straight.

How did you feel? What sensations did you have as you moved your legs in this way, compared to the way you did it earlier? How does your back feel, your neck? and your head? Is there some difference?

You could do this three more times. Always move gently, easily, giving your mental directions while thinking of the invisible puppeteer moving one knee up and then the other, or sliding one heel down the floor and then the other. Moving your legs this way can give you a rather delicious sensation in your limbs and in your back.

When you move in this way, with your mind guiding your body, your whole body can feel different as you lie on the table. See for yourself how you feel now: do you feel longer, smoother, more relaxed? That is lengthening.

Now that you have directed more length into yourself, it is important that you come to standing in a way that will not interfere with this additional length. Use the way that you have learned earlier in this book: gently bend one knee and then the other, and leaving your knees bent, roll your head to one side; let your whole body follow the head and roll over; continue rolling over until you are on your hands and knees and then gently stand on one foot; from there come all the way up to standing. Continue leaving your chin lowered and looking down until you are standing, and then gently let your eyes come to eye level and let your head follow. Can you feel the additional lengthening, ease and lightness in your body as you stand and walk?

▶ Abbreviating the Directions

I myself went through several stages with the mental directions. When I was a beginning student, I used to say all three complete phrases, "Let the neck be free, to let the head go forward and up, to let the back lengthen and widen." After a while, I eliminated the words "let the."

You may want to eliminate the word "let," as I did, but it would be a mistake to do this immediately. The word "let" is important. It means "allow." Let or allow means you do not *do* anything, you merely *permit it to happen*. After a period of using the phrases in their entirety, you find that you automatically *allow*, and the word "let" is no longer required. The directions could now be abbreviated to: "Neck free. Head forward and up. Back lengthen and widen."

These are the words I then said to myself, over and over, not only while I was at my Alexander lessons, but also while walking in the street, sitting at my office desk, bending, and anything else I did. It would not be an audible whisper. You would not see my lips move as if I were talking to myself. I said the words mentally.

Saying words mentally brings an instant response. Messages go from the brain to the muscles via the nervous system at a speed close to the speed of light. The speed is so fast that the message is received by the muscles even before we finish thinking the words or the phrase. The Alexander student is never asked to "concentrate" on the words or to mouth them laboriously, as this interferes with the remarkable speed with which the messages are transmitted.

Say them rapidly, lightly.

Then, as I did, you might shorten the procedure again. I eventually found that when I said the words, "head forward and up," instantly my neck muscles and back muscles responded without my having to mention those parts specifically. I could also say only the world "lengthen" or "neck free." The muscular reaction was the same for me as if I had said all the Alexander directions.

"Lengthen" became the word that worked best for me. It became, for me, the whole concept of the neck releasing and the head going forward and up, as well as the back lengthening and widening.

Then came a stage where, by simply becoming aware that I was tense or starting to tense, I instantly released. I did not have to mentally say the words at all.

This was the *most subtle* "directing" of all. It came about after some months.

Whenever I started a new activity, I used the full Alexander directions. For instance, one winter I took up skiing. The new experience of the difficulty of keeping my balance on the skis caused me to "tighten up." This made matters worse. My old habits of swaying my lower back, tightening the back of my neck and pulling my shoulders forward appeared to return with this new experience, although only slightly. It was enough to make me feel that I was a clumsy ball of tension. I remembered my Alexander directions, and I said them in full.

I realized that on skis I had a lot of anxiety about falling and hurting myself. The words worked. My body released the tension; I gained my balance and I gained my confidence. From then on, I learned rapidly.

As you use the Alexander directions in your life and you have found that they can be abbreviated with good results, remember that any stressful activity is likely to require a lengthening of the phrases in order to revive the lengthening of your back. And you may find that certain constant activities require more direction than others.

One woman, 53, with rheumatoid arthritis since the age of 15, had great improvement from her Alexander lessons. However, in damp weather she was in more pain and felt she could not get out of bed or out of a chair. She then reminded herself of the three directions and was able to get up. Or, she would stand at the foot of a flight of stairs, unable to begin the climb, having become rigid from fear of pain. She would give herself the full directions and up she went, step by step as she continued to repeat the words. She added that she felt that she "floated upwards." Her family corroborated this.

Alexander himself had no one to give him the directions. He gave them to himself. You can do likewise. But remember, it took great perseverance by Alexander over a long period of time to gain his full joy.

▶ What The Directions Mean And How They Work

The whole idea of the Alexander Technique is to help people "come out" of a condition in their bodies that is compressing, tightening, and shortening them. This downward pull in the muscles is the target of the Alexander directions. Extra downward pull means extra contraction. Extra contraction is a load on the body against which it must eventually protest. You can feel this contraction in exaggerated fashion merely by slumping.

You are probably already sitting in a somewhat slumped position—unless you are an Alexander student—so in order to feel this contraction, you need to exaggerate the slump. Do it now. Slump way down. Sit on the middle of a chair and let your shoulders and back slump down. Exaggerate. Now notice how your body is. Notice your neck, your shoulders, your back, your abdomen.

Can you sense that the back of your neck has shortened and tightened? And has it pulled your head backwards? Check on this by dropping the chin slightly and see how the back of the neck releases. Tighten the back of your neck again and notice how it shortens, and pulls your head backwards. Your chin is now jutting out ahead of you.

It is the tightening of the muscles in the back of your neck that pulls your head into an unnatural position, which in turn reinforces the shortening (or contraction) of the neck, back and spine. Many of you do this all the time, in all activities, and are now experiencing an exaggeration of your usual habits.

To allow your head to go forward where it really belongs and to allow the back to regain its length, you need to release the back of your neck. Do it now. Release the back of your neck. Let it be free. Notice that as you do so, you allow your chin to lower and your neck

SITTING

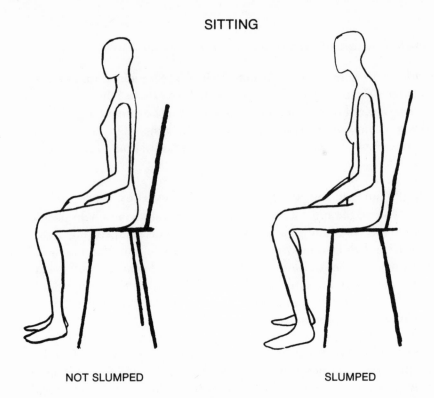

NOT SLUMPED   SLUMPED

gets longer. See how this brings your head into a more forward position.

You have just experienced "Let the neck be free."

To restore more lengthening to your back, tell your head to go up in tiny steps or increments. Do this now. Let your head *actually* move upwards a tiny bit at a time, following your thoughts. Notice how, while your neck is free and your head is going forward and upward, your spine and back become more upright. You gradually come out of your slump.

Do only as much as feels comfortable and easy. See if you can sense that the length is coming from inside you, as you say the thoughts to yourself. Let your mind lead your body, and let your head follow your mind. See if you can sense when the moment has come to leave it alone, to not do any more upward movement, no matter how gentle it may seem to you. See if you can sense that if you do one more little movement upwards, it would be a little too much work, a little too much tension, instead of the normal amount of tension that is required to bring you upwards and maintain you there. You may continue to give your Alexander directions. If you like, you can try this again. You can slump down again and use your Alexander directions to bring you up, always thinking of your head leading; allow your head to make these very small movements upwards and allow your neck and torso to float upwards into more length following your lead.

In this instance, I have asked you to *actually* move your head a little bit, because you had made yourself slump more than you habitually do. To undo the additional slumping and pulling down, you needed to do a slight muscular movement of going upwards to counteract it.

The whole procedure of coming out of the slump was initiated by the lengthening in the back of your neck. When you "let the neck be free," you freed the rest of your body.

Although the Alexander directions are in three phrases, it all happens at once as the neck becomes free. As you let the neck be free, you are simultaneously letting the head come forward and up and the back to lengthen and widen. The changes in the head and back cannot happen until you release your neck. When you release your neck, your head and back respond simultaneously.

"Say the words all together one after the other," as Alexander used to say. Physically we cannot say these words all together. We are compelled to say them one after the other. You can realize for yourself, though, that as the words come out in sequence, the body responds as one unit.

Alexander directions bring about a learning on a deep level. The body learns in a way in which it is learning all the time, but more rapidly; and, of course, it is learning good rather than bad use. This manner of learning takes only minutes. Reinforcement is necessary, through repetition. A taste of the joy is experienced at the beginning, and the reinforcement permits the joy to become complete and lasting.

The level of learning via the Alexander teaching is at nerve and cell level. This is quite different than a mechanical type of learning such as that which takes place when we say, "Stand up straight," or "Stand against the wall and push your back against the wall." You may learn to stand straight in this way, but this approach is both superficial and artificial compared to the depth of learning effected by the Alexander Technique. Forcing does not integrate "standing straight" within the cells, nerves, and muscles of the body. It does not become—as it does through the Alexander Technique—second nature. It is as forced and unnatural as a suit of armor. Some people have developed neck or back pain, or both, from locking themselves into this suit of armor. Wilhelm Reich saw muscular tension and blocking as "armoring" which also blocked emotional freedom and joy.

▶ Sitting-To-Standing, and Standing Up

In the first chapter, when the whole concept of giving yourself "directions" was new, we did a sitting-to-standing movement with Alexander directions. Now that these directions are more familiar to you and how they work is better understood, you may experience an increased sensation of lightness as you again go through the sitting-to-standing movement. Let us try it.

Sit on the middle of your chair, not too close to the edge to be uncomfortable. Your back is not in contact with the back of the chair. Sit naturally, without trying to be straight.

Tell the back of your neck to be free. Tell those muscles to release. Allow your forehead to move a little forward, by permitting your chin to lower slightly. (Do *not* move your neck forward. Your neck is directed *upwards*.)

Tell your head that it is moving upwards toward the ceiling. Tell it to float upwards in small movements. While you are continuously permitting your chin to lower and thinking of your head floating upwards, gently move your head and torso slightly forward in the chair and *allow yourself* to move up out of the chair, still thinking of your head floating up to the ceiling and leading your body upwards.

When you are standing, continue the thought: "Head forward and up, back lengthening." Remain standing.

You have perhaps just experienced getting up out of a chair effortlessly. Now that you are standing, check out your back. What do your lower back and buttocks feel like? Do you find that you have tightened them at the very end of the process, as you rose to your feet?

Do your legs also feel tight? Have you thrown your shoulders back somewhat, or have you let them slump downwards?

If you have done any one or more of these things, it means that you worked hard at the end of the movement to try and finish the process of standing up in the way that you usually do.

Now tell the back of your neck to be free. Allow your head to move slightly forward and the chin to drop slightly lower. And tell your head that it is floating upwards in small movements toward the ceiling. Be aware of the changes in your body. Have the buttocks dropped slightly and become less tense? Has this released tension in your legs, back and shoulders?

STANDING

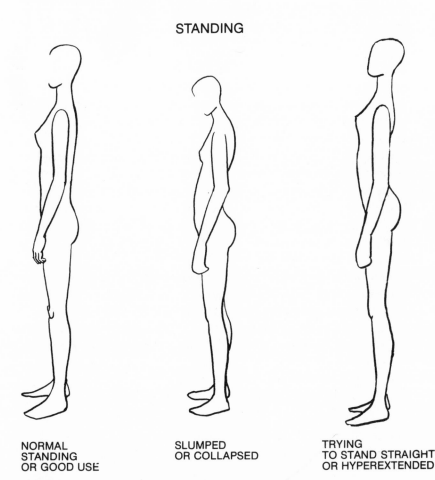

NORMAL
STANDING
OR GOOD USE

SLUMPED
OR COLLAPSED

TRYING
TO STAND STRAIGHT
OR HYPEREXTENDED

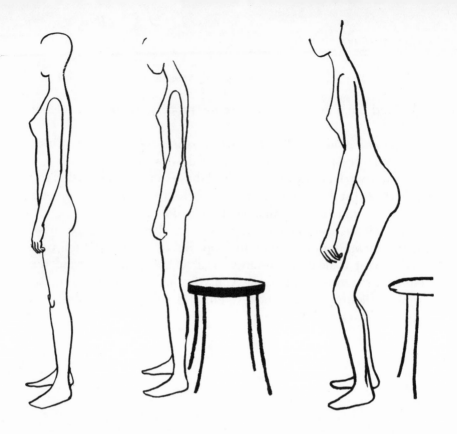

Let us use these same directions to return to a sitting position.

Stand in front of the chair. Read the instructions, put the book down, and follow the directions.

Allow your chin to drop slightly, permitting your forehead to go forward. *Tell your head that it is floating upwards* in small movements toward the ceiling. It is going forward and up toward a spot on the ceiling not exactly above you, but a few inches forward of that. *While continuing that thought*, gradually *let* your knees bend and your hip joints bend, until your buttocks meet the chair.

Did this feel easier and more familiar to you now than when you did it in the first chapter? Do you feel that after having been reading about neck free, head forward and up, back lengthening, through these chapters, there may have been some effect on you?

Use your directions again to come up to standing. This time let us learn from the previous time. DO NOT FINISH STANDING UP.

As soon as your legs have unbent, and are straight (*not* locked), you *are* standing up, even though you may not feel erect. You are not falling down and you are not sitting down. You are standing up. You

STANDING TO SITTING

GOOD USE

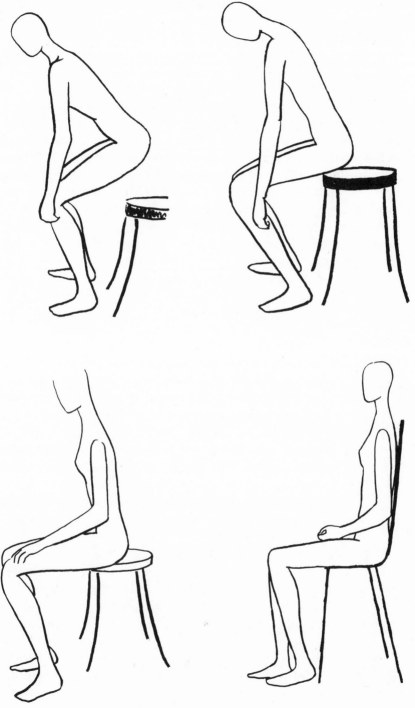

may not *feel* erect; it is quite likely that you feel as if the upper half of your torso is leaning forward. You need a mirror to show you what is really going on in your body as your feelings are not reliable, just as Alexander discovered that *his* feelings were not reliable.

Move your chair near a mirror so that when you sit on the chair you would be able to see your profile in the mirror. You would, of course, need to turn your head to one side to see your profile. After looking in the mirror at your profile, come up to standing with your Alexander directions, and see if you can do it without "finishing" standing up. Now look in the mirror at your profile, by gently turning your head, and see whether you are standing up straight.

As I had said earlier, our feelings are unreliable. When we have been accustomed to standing with a sway back, that is what feels straight to us. When you stand without that sway back, you do *not* feel straight, even though your back may be much straighter without that sway in the middle. Ironically, when people *try* to stand up straight, they create even more of a sway back, as in the drawing shown.

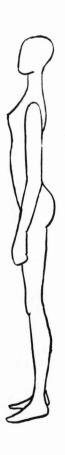

This is a very difficult part of the process of standing, to arrive without straining the back, and also to not be slumped down. It is difficult because you are not used to it and do not know what it really feels like, and therefore you cannot recognize the feeling when you have it; you are likely to say, "No, that's wrong! I'm not standing straight at all!" and then you will do something that *feels straight* to you and is actually making your back arch. I do not promise that you can find this on your own. With perseverance and a great deal of painstaking observation in the mirror you may eventually find it for yourself, as Alexander did.

The ideal would be to use a three-way mirror, which Alexander himself did. Otherwise, each time you turn your head, you could be pulling your neck down and your head backwards and downwards. More learning is required to know how to turn your head without interfering with the length in your body. With a three-way mirror, you can see your profile without turning your head and you have a truer picture of your profile.

In sitting, there is the same difficulty as in standing, that our feelings are unreliable. With most of us, when we feel we are sitting straight, there is actually an arch in our backs, or a sway back, and when we are actually straight, we feel that we are a little slumped over. I would like to help you through words to come to know the difference between lengthening and contracting while sitting.

Sit on your chair and gently turn your head towards the mirror so that you can see your profile. Are you curved backwards? Or is there a forward curve in the middle of your back, which is the equivalent of a sway back? Look at the drawings and see whether it is one or the other of these curves that you see in the mirror. Now try to straighten up, and look again in the mirror, and I think you will see that now you definitely have a strong curvature in the middle of your back: your belly protrudes forward at the same time, and your hip bones are protruding forward.

I would like you to talk to your hip bones and tell them to gently go

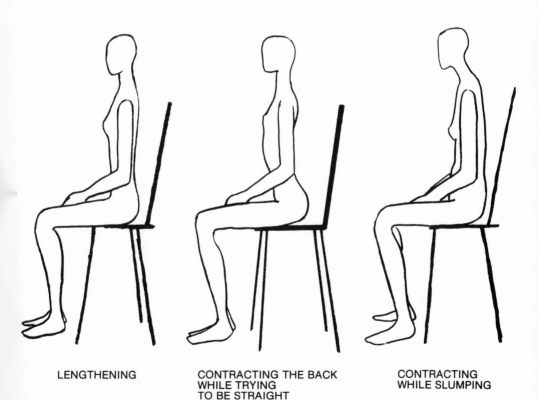

LENGTHENING   CONTRACTING THE BACK   CONTRACTING
                           WHILE TRYING   WHILE SLUMPING
                           TO BE STRAIGHT

a little bit backwards. As you talk to them, allow them to follow your words, and allow them to go backwards *slightly*. Do this while your head is facing front, not staring, with your chin slightly lowered, and with Alexander upward directions. When you have allowed your hips to go back a little bit, gently turn your head to the side and look in the mirror; is there less of that curve in the middle of your back? Or perhaps it no longer exists? You probably feel that your back is not straight; you probably feel that it is now curved in the opposite direction. You can tell from this how unreliable your feelings are. When you thought you were straight, your back was curved, pushing your hipbones forwards; when you allow your back to be erect, with ease, then you feel that your back is curved in the opposite direction, as if you have pushed your hips too far backward.

We need to reeducate our feelings as well as our bodies. I suggest that you do this sometimes in front of the mirror until you get to know what is more erect; eventually you can reach a stage when what you feel is the same as what you see in the mirror. When you gently allow your hips to go backwards what you are doing is putting a stop to keeping them forwards. When you stop holding the hip bones forward, they will come into their natural place and your whole torso becomes lengthened and straighter.

Without the mirror, you can use your hand to give you feedback. Very gently move one hand and slide it *very lightly* up and down your back to tell you what is going on there. You need to be careful though that when you move your hand you let it float to your back and touch it as lightly as a feather; otherwise, if you put a lot of effort into moving your hand you will jerk your arm backwards and throw your whole back into a twist. The idea is to leave your back alone, and gently move your hand backwards to touch it very lightly. After you have slid your hand up and down your middle and lower back two or three times you can tell what your back is doing, whether it is straight, or whether it is curved. If it is curved, you may talk to your body and allow it to come into the position that feels straighter to your hand; do it with ease, gentleness, and *very delicately. Delicacy is the key to the Alexander Technique.*

If you wish, you could do as Alexander did and perseveringly work in front of a three-way mirror to improve yourself. It took Alexander many years, and he was a brilliant man. So you can expect it to take a very long time when you work on your own, as well as almost inhuman patience. And you may or may not succeed.

If you are not willing to take this route, and it is without a guarantee of success, I suggest an alternate way to work on your own. Observe yourself once or twice sitting and standing in front of a mirror, preferably a three-way mirror, and then walk away from the mirror. For the rest of the day, instead of practicing in front of the mirror, apply the directions and your new awareness during those times in your daily life when you sit and stand.

➤ Changes in Your Perception

The Alexander Technique focuses strongly on sitting and standing. Although repeated again and again, it does not become tedious. The student experiences different sensations. The student changes. As the change in movement occurs it is accompanied by a change in feeling. Both the movement and the feeling become more and more pleasurable.

This repetition of simple movements with simple directions can be good news to the reader who wishes to attain at least a sampling of Alexander joy. Projected through your own repeated experience, it can lead to higher and higher levels of pleasure.

I repeat: you will not be enjoying the benefits of an Alexander lesson. But you *can* be experiencing improvement as your body responds to your directions. You might think that you would enjoy playing a flute. But until you take lessons, you cannot even imagine the enjoyment that flute playing can bring.

Repeat the directions. Give yourself the directions while sitting and standing, over and over. Enjoy. You will feel as though you are beginning to have a different body. The repetition will not be tedious as this evolving body of yours begins to "pay off" in new delight from many unexpected directions.

I have often had a student say to me after several lessons, "Oh, you are teaching me differently now." It has seemed different to them because they themselves have changed. I am teaching them in exactly the same way. Sometimes they say, "Oh, we never did this movement before," when actually we had gone through that movement in every lesson. It is as if they have a different body.

It will begin to feel differently to you, too, as you reach new levels of body awareness and greater degrees of good body use. You will be encouraged to continue doing what you are doing, using these simple procedures. The benefits snowball through repetition. Repetition changes habits.

We all have one problem in common: the need to work with gravity. Going up from sitting to standing provides the experience of going up against gravity. Going down from standing to sitting is the experience of going down with gravity. The strain of getting to a standing position or of keeping ourselves from flopping or falling into a sitting position is an ideal living experience to work with. Succeed in the gravity struggle of sitting and standing and you can succeed in all of the secondary gravity confronting movements.

You begin to use your body in the best way, no matter what you do with it, with greater ease.

You have taken almost all of your life to "learn" the wrong use of your body. You have formed unnatural habits by repetition. Through the Alexander Technique you are not really learning new habits, you are "unlearning" unwanted habits and relearning what you once knew.

➤ A Sitting and Standing Exercise

I have shown you how you can help yourself in sitting and standing with Alexander directions and with a greater awareness of how you use yourself. I would like now to share with you a simple exercise that could enhance the whole process.

The difference between an exercise and an "Alexander experience" is that an exercise cannot be done during your everyday activities, while your "Alexander experiences" can be applied to your daily life. An exercise, however, can help you when you are on your own, and lead to a more heightened sense of change.

Sit on the chair fairly close to the edge of the chair. Not too close to the edge, or you will feel that you are going to fall off the chair. Stand up and sit down two or three times, in the way that is most natural for you. Notice, as you did in the first chapter, what this feels like; how does it feel in your neck, your back, your thighs, and your feet? Now stay seated on the chair. Sit with your legs comfortably apart, with your feet placed under and below your knees, so that when you look down you can see that your knees are poised over your feet. I would like you to leave your legs and feet apart while you go through the movements I am going to show you. These movements will help you improve sitting down and standing up.

While you are sitting on the chair, move both knees right and left as a small, gentle movement, five or six times. This is to experience the legs being free and moving freely at the hip joints. After a few times, let your legs come back to the middle.

This time, move your knees in and out, in towards each other, and out away from each other. Do this movement a few times; it is a simple, easy movement of moving the knees lightly in and out. You may do it playfully, as fun. After a few times let your legs come to the middle.

How do your legs feel, and your hip joints, and your back?

Now sway your head and torso right and left. Small easy movements, playful movements. Let your head and torso move as one piece, right and left. Now you are experiencing your torso moving separately from your legs. Your legs do not move now, only your torso is moving. These movements give you the experience of the separation between your torso and your legs, and the separation is at the hip joints. After you have moved your head and torso five or six times, from side to side, let your torso come to rest in the middle. Take stock here, for a few seconds, and notice how you are sitting on the chair. Does anything feel different in your legs, or your hip joints, or your back, or your neck, or your shoulders? Does anything feel easier in the way you are sitting on the chair now?

Now do a small, gentle movement, moving your torso forwards and backwards; stay within the range of comfort, not too far forwards, and not too far backwards. It is better to do a smaller movement than a larger movement. Do small, gentle movements forwards and backwards, your head and torso moving together.

As you continue doing this movement, I would like you to gradually increase the size of the movement and gradually go further forwards and further backwards. Each time you do the movement, go a little bit further than the time before. Please *increase it only gradually*. Do only a little bit more than the time before, until eventually you are doing rather large movements, swaying forwards and backwards. Continue these large movements and the next time you go forward, allow yourself to continue the forward movement to come up to standing, and then come to sitting on the chair again and swing backwards; then swing far forwards, and upwards to standing. Continue doing the movement like this a few times, so that you experience coming up to standing as a continuation of moving forwards, and the continuation is moving forwards and upwards.

After you have done this a few times, I would like you to do it again, and this time, when you move forwards, and start moving upwards to standing, notice at which point you feel a tension in your legs, back, neck, or thighs. At that point, freeze in that position. Now continue moving upwards to standing, and see if the movement was not smoother and easier when you continued.

Come to sitting again. Do the movement this way two or three times so that each time you move forwards and up to standing, at the moment you feel the tightening of any muscles, you stop. Freeze in that position for one or two seconds, and then continue your motion forwards and upwards to standing. I think you will find that it becomes smoother and easier, and you have eliminated the tension.

After you have done that about three more times, stay seated on your chair with your legs and feet comfortably apart, your knees poised over your feet. See whether sitting on the chair has improved or changed in any way. Does sitting feel easier than the last time that you took stock?

With your right hand, take hold of a piece of your hair on the top of your head and swing forwards and backwards, starting with small movements. Think that your hand holding the hair is guiding and directing your movements so that instead of an Alexander teacher moving you forwards and backwards, your own hand is doing it for you through the help of your hair. *Do not pull hard* on your hair; I don't want you to hurt yourself, or pull out a chunk of hair. Instead, you can pull very lightly and gently on your hair, just enough to feel that it is guiding you and moving you. When your movements become large, allow your hand to gently pull your hair forwards and upwards to standing; and come down to sitting again. Do this a few times, and see whether there is any difference when you have your hand guiding you. After a few times, change hands. Do it with your left hand. First, do small movements forwards and backwards with your hand holding your hair and guiding you. Then allow the movement to become larger until you feel that it is perfectly natural to follow through to standing—that coming to standing is a continuation of moving forwards, and do this two or three times with your left hand holding your hair.

Is there a difference between using your right hand holding your hair or your left hand? After you have done this about three times, come back to your chair and let go of your hair. Check yourself again. How do you feel while sitting? Does your back feel straighter? More upright? Does it feel easier? Less tense? Does your neck feel freer? Do your thighs feel freer? Do your legs feel easier? Does your head feel that it is poised more lightly on the tip of your spine? Maybe it feels as if it is floating towards the ceiling.

Let us do this movement a little differently. Take another chair and place it in front of the chair that you are sitting on, and lightly place your hands on the back of the chair in front of you. Sit fairly close to the edge of your chair, legs comfortably apart, as you did before. With your hands resting lightly on the chair in front of you, gently sway forwards and backwards a little; *gradually* let that movement become larger and larger, then let the movement continue up to standing. And come to sitting again.

Leave your hands on the back of the chair in front of you, touching lightly. Swing backwards, and as you swing forwards *think* of lifting your bottom off the chair and you will find that you have come to standing. Now that you are standing, you need to find a way to sitting. Your hands may have left the chair in front of you. Place your hands on the back of the chair. You will do the reverse of the movement that you did to come to standing. With your hands lightly touching the back of the chair, start to bend at the knees and hips joints, and move your bottom downwards towards the chair. Then you swing backwards, and as you swing forwards, you let your bottom rise up in the air, looking downwards with your eyes, and you have come to standing; allow your knees and hip joints to bend, and allow your bottom to float down to the chair. Think of your bottom floating upwards and floating downwards, and see how standing and sitting feels to you now, as you do it this way. Do this three or four more times, and then stay on the chair. Remove the chair in front of you.

Let us see now what it is like to simply stand up and sit down. Do it normally, and see if it has changed. Do you feel more integrated? Do your joints feel better oiled? Do you feel that your back is more integrated with your neck and your head? Do you feel that your legs are moving more freely and are moving as something separate from your torso and your head?

Rest on the chair for a short while. When you are rested, sit and stand with your Alexander directions. Has that added something more of lightness and ease? Perhaps you feel that it has never been so easy.

During these movements, which are from one of Dr. Feldenkrais' lessons, I have never really asked you to think of standing up or sitting down. It is the same as in an Alexander lesson, where we ask our students *not* to think of standing up or sitting down. Instead of an Alexander teacher taking you up and down, I have asked you to use certain thoughts to help you come to standing, and to sitting. I have also asked you to do certain movements, that are not part of your daily life, that help you come to standing and sitting more easily. In this way, you have given yourself the experience of having your body function with lengthening and lightness, with the head going forward and up and the neck being free, and the back lengthening. Perhaps from now on standing and sitting will be a different experience for you, easier, more akin to the Alexander way of moving.

If you did find improvement in the way you sit and stand after this experiment then this shows you that it was very effective to use a way that is indirect, a way that eliminates the poor habits you usually use. When you eliminate poor habits, then you have good use. This exercise was a demonstration of that, showing you that you got the improvement fairly rapidly, in a matter of minutes, not hours or weeks. You improved your standing and sitting without having tried to improve it directly, without practicing the same movement in the same way each time. When we try to improve a movement directly, we are likely to tighten up, work too hard, and work against ourselves. We *impose* more tension, and work; a far more effective means is to find ways to eliminate the hard work, and then we can re-experience the natural, easy joyous flow of good movement!

➡ Walking with Direction

I believe it is easier to flow into walking from a sitting position, rather than from standing. I always prefer to use the easier way to initiate learning. When you use the easy way, before you know it the more difficult way has also become easy, without practice.

First, let us try an experiment. Sit on a chair and stand up and walk around the room in the way you usually do, without trying to improve any part of it.

Now, sit on a chair and slump down. Remain slumped down as you stand up and walk around the room. Really slump!

See what it does to your legs, and your butt. I think you will sense your legs as tighter and heavier, and your butt more constricted and pushed downwards; and your feet land more heavily on the floor. Can you sense the tightness in the back of your neck and shoulders, and all the way down your back?

Now walk in your usual way and compare. You may be doing the same things as when you were slumping down, only to a lesser degree. See if you can recognize what your poor habits of use are as you walk.

Now use your Alexander directions to bring you upwards into more length and more lightness; the essence of it is to think of your head leading your torso upwards, and to allow your head to be slightly forward by lowering your chin slightly. The change is to be very slight, very delicate. See if you can become aware when you start to push yourself upwards, which is what I do *not* want you to do. It is almost inevitable that you will start to push yourself upwards now and again, even though it may be subtle. When you feel yourself doing that, stop pushing, aand think of lengthening. Do you feel easier now?

Again, walk around in a slump and compare the differences.

I would like now to give you some additional helpful directions for walking and see if you can have even more of the "Alexander experience" in this activity than you have had so far. Let us start the easy way, by sitting on a chair.

Using your awareness and your Alexander directions, come from sitting to standing, allowing your body to remain soft while directing length lightly. Think again of your head floating gently forward and upward—perhaps you will actually feel a slight lightening and lengthening in yourself. As you direct your head forwards and upwards and your back to lengthen and widen, *allow* one knee to lift and bend slightly and begin to walk. As you walk and direct, lower your chin slightly and let your eyes look *downwards into the far distance*. Your eyes are neither looking down at your feet, nor straining to look at eye level or higher.

You need not be careful as you walk; *walk as if you haven't a care in the world* or as if you are taking your dog out for a stroll. Do *not* try to walk differently than you usually do with your legs. *Let your walk be natural*, and *direct lightly*: neck free, head going forward and up, back lengthening and widening. Stop for a second. Direct yourself again while standing still: say the thoughts two or three times. The next time you say them, slightly lift and bend one knee and begin to walk. As you walk, you could even say to yourself: "I am not going to think about walking, I will think instead of my head going up and my back lengthening." Several times, after a few steps, stand in one place and direct lightly, and then resume your "well-directed" walk; *each time lower your chin slightly again and look softly into the distance*.

I have observed in my students that initially, even when they start walking with good direction, after two or three steps the old tight habits start creeping into their bodies, always involving the back of the neck tightening. Stopping after every few steps brings a halt to the poor habits, and you are free to redirect and reexperience a few more steps of walking with good direction.

An excellent direction for walking is to think of your *weight going upwards*. When people walk, their weight tends to shift from one foot to the other, from side to side, and this is eliminated by directing your weight upwards. This direction can replace the other directions, or, you may find it more fun to alternate between "head forward and up" and "weight going upwards."

Walk towards a mirror without directing yourself and see if you notice yourself swaying slightly from side to side as you walk; or you might see one foot coming down heavily, then the other. Walk again toward the mirror *with* your directions, and perhaps you will see yourself walking more smoothly, almost gliding.

Legs and feet move better when you are directing your head and back. It usually is not helpful to *try* and change what your feet and legs are doing; this causes more strain, which can reach all the way up the back to the neck. Instead, as you lighten the weight of your head and torso, the burden on your legs is released, and your leg and feet muscles are automatically freer. A great deal of the contraction that has pulled your legs and feet out of their good, natural alignment is released. The legs and feet move better—straighter, and with more ease.

Can you sense how your natural flexibility has a chance to be functioning when your downward pulls are prevented?

I would like to restate how to experience an improvement in your walking: start by sitting on a chair and *allow walking to be a continuation of the sitting-to-standing motion;* while walking, stop after every few steps *to recapture good direction.*

➡️ All Movement Becomes the Act of Lengthening

I would like to propose a novel way of thinking of your body movements. I would like you to think that *all activities are the same thing. They are all one action: the action of lengthening.*

Standing is not different from sitting, and sitting is not different from walking, and walking is not different from standing. The activity is LENGTHENING and your body *happens* to go through different motions while lengthening.

I think you will be far more successful if you do not think of sitting as being different from standing and standing as being different from walking. Do not think of going from one movement to another. *They are all one and the same—all movement is neck free, head forward and up, back lengthening and widening.* Standing still is the same as lying down, and lying down is the same as walking; it is all LENGTHENING.

Let your mind focus—gently— on LENGTHENING and the rest will take care of itself.

And here is a reminder: that LENGTHENING involves the whole concept of the head leading upward and the neck and torso gently lengthening upwards following the head. As the neck and torso are attached to the head, they have no choice but to follow the head. *Please do not try to make* your head go upwards; simply give the mental order in your mind, and mentally be aware that the neck and back are also lengthening.

Now you may be ready for another experience: to start walking from a standing position.

I do not recommend "practicing" this unless you feel that there is some improvement in your standing posture or alignment. The major improvement would be the feeling that it feels *easy* to be standing. Another improvement would be in your image in the mirror—a long, smooth, back and neck, and straighter legs; again, as I so often stress—*without any feeling of effort or strain*. It always helps, in almost every activity, to lower your chin slightly while "directing upwards."

From this "well-directed" standing, you move gently into walking by lowering your chin slightly more (do *not* lower your neck), looking down in the distance, directing yourself upwards, and allowing one knee to move, then the other, without thinking of your knees. All this can take place in an instant; it should not be time-consuming.

Once you have allowed your legs to move, *do not think of your legs*. They have been "walking" you for a lifetime and know how to do it. You can trust them to get you where you want to go. Direct your head, neck and back upwards, and automatically your legs become free to move with ease.

Instead of aiming for your destination, *think of aiming for the ceiling*.

By consciously giving yourself the directions while sitting, standing or walking, you can magnify the good effects many times. *Give the thoughts as you go through the day*.

➡ A New Way of Thinking

You are on your own now. I have told you how to direct yourself while lying down, sitting, standing and walking.

One of the most important realizations that I have had about the

Alexander Technique is that it is NOT teaching you how to sit, stand and walk. *You know how to do that.*

THE ALEXANDER TECHNIQUE IS TEACHING YOU HOW TO *THINK.*

All your life you have been sitting, standing and walking. Count the number of years you have been doing it. You may not be doing it in the best and easiest way, but you know how to do it.

What I am teaching you is how to think as you do your activities of life. *When your thinking improves, your actions improve.*

I am teaching you to avoid *thinking down* (as in "sitting down" or "bending down") or of *getting up*, or of being straight.

The Alexander Technique is simple: the basic concept is "lengthening," which refers to the muscles of your body. However, you are not always going to be directing up to the ceiling. After all, sometimes you are lying down and not going in the direction of the ceiling. When bending, you are also not going to the ceiling, and I will teach you in the next chapter how to direct while bending.

In my sixteen years of teaching, I have had two students who were creating new pain in their body in between their lessons. After some "cross-examination" on my part, I discovered that they were thinking of lengthening "downwards." As soon as it became clear to them that the lengthening went *up the body*, presto, no more pain.

You need to be very accurate in what you are thinking.

Others have created discomfort by *trying to do* the directions. You cannot possibly make your head reach the ceiling—so why try? *Let it happen in your mind.*

You are on your own with your directions, without a teacher. Should you feel pain or discomfort while carrying out my suggestions, you are probably doing one of two things:

a) you are *directing yourself downwards, or thinking downwards;* you may be thinking of your feet or your legs or of pulling your buttocks under, and that is sufficient to cause a contraction in your whole body that can bring about discomfort, aching, and even pain;

b) *you are trying to make yourself go upwards;* you may be *trying* to push your head upwards, or you may be *trying* to free your neck or push it backwards, or you may be *trying* to make your back straight.

Just as an Alexander teacher needs to think of the lengthening, and not try to do anything for the student, so you need to do the same when teaching yourself. Many people find it hard to believe that *doing nothing and only thinking upwards* can do anything for them. TRUST THE DIRECTIONS, TRUST THE NONDOING, TRUST THE ALEXANDER TECHNIQUE.

If you are not willing to have this trust, you cannot possibly get the benefits. I realize that I am proposing very different ways of learning and of doing things that are contrary to our education. However, when you continue to do things the way you have always done them, how can you change? You need to know how to *stop* doing the things in the way you are used to, the way that has seemed right to you for so long, and then you can experience a change. That is NONDOING.

Even without a teacher you will receive immense dividends for every mental direction you give yourself while sitting, standing, walking.

PLEASURE IS THE KEY. The pleasure principle is an important factor in permanent learning. Whether you give yourself directions alone or take an Alexander lesson, the whole process needs to be pleasurable. We automatically want to maintain anything that is pleasurable, and get rid of anything that is not. Since it is not strenuous, we are not tiring the nervous system so it can readily continue to absorb and integrate the experience. The message circulates between the muscles, nervous system and brain, and then back again to the nervous system and the muscles. The gist of the message is, "I like this. This feels very nice. I want to keep this feeling."

➡ Some Peculiar Feelings That Are Possible

An interesting thing happens frequently in Alexander work. Students often feel strange, especially in the beginning. *They feel relaxed, and also "peculiar."* For instance, when a student is first experiencing standing, after coming up out of a chair with the teacher's help and using the Alexander directions, he often feels that he is not standing up straight. He feels as if he is leaning forward from the waist with the upper torso. It takes a look in the mirror to convince him that he is really not bending over and that his posture is erect. He begins to understand that what felt straight to him before must have been somewhat less than erect.

The way you normally stand feels straight to you and any change from that will feel peculiar. You have looked at yourself in a full length mirror, viewing your profile by slowly turning your head without twisting your body. You saw a person with a certain figure. It could have been an "S" curve or a straight "I" or anything in-between.

When you give yourself Alexander directions, a change takes place. At first, that change may feel "abnormal." When the "abnormal" begins to feel normal, you realize that it was the way in which you were previously standing that was really not right.

If you have been doing the Alexander experiences and the Feldenkrais exercises as you progressed through these chapters, you may want to look in that same mirror again and see what changes have taken place by now in your profile.

Here is a simple demonstration of how peculiar an unfamiliar feeling can be. Clasp your hands together with the fingers intertwined. Notice which thumb is closest to you, right or left. Now unclasp and then reclasp your hands with the other thumb in front.

How does this feel? For most people, it feels "wrong." It feels comparable to shaking hands with your left hand. It feels peculiar because you have made a change from your habitual way. Some members of your family may clasp their hands left thumb in front, some with right thumb in front. Were they all to be asked to clasp their hands right thumb in front, the left-thumb claspers would feel peculiar about it, whereas the right-thumb claspers would feel the position to be perfectly natural.

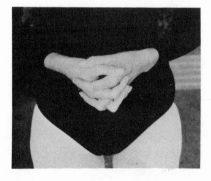 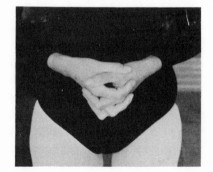

I point out this "peculiar feeling" syndrome, because if you are working on your own, you could be wrongly discouraged by it. Of course, working with the Alexander teacher, you will be given an explanation and encouragement.

If you feel peculiar, use your mirror to confirm that there is no real basis for this feeling and that you are making changes for the better. Later it will feel normal, and then if you should imitate the way you used to stand, *that* will feel peculiar.

Often, a person taking Alexander lessons feels "wrong" in the first lessons, and only when looking in the mirror and seeing that it is not the way he felt is he convinced all is right with himself. The most clear example of this is with the shoulders. Many people have one shoulder lower than the other. During Alexander lessons, as a result of the "lengthening and widening", the shoulders may become level. A person who had the right shoulder lower than the left to start with would now feel that the right shoulder is too high. The mirror would show him that the shoulders are level. After one or two more experiences like this with his teacher, the level shoulders come to *feel level* to the student. The reeducation has taken place.

With a teacher, the reeducation of the feelings happens quite fast; on your own, it will take longer.

▶ A Valuable Dividend Of Body Awareness

For most people, the directing of attention to the body in ways we have been discussing and experiencing is a new focus for consciousness. Our consciousness, when directed to the body, is usually sense-oriented. We treat our body to tastes, odors and tactile pleasures. Seldom do we examine our body as intensely as we have now been doing and rarely are we as aware of how our body feels.

This body awareness pays off. The Alexander student who may have been hunching his shoulders up toward his ears, and who is now enjoying a more natural place, may get into a stressful situation where momentarily the shoulders tend to regress to an old habit. Thanks to a new body awareness, the moment that this happens, the Alexander student becomes aware of it. Even if the shoulders tense only slightly, the student is immediately conscious of it.

Being aware of it prevents the shoulders from going any further into a hunched position and may even cause the shoulders to return to the normal position. This would be the case for an advanced student. More than likely the Alexander student will want to give himself the directions, "Neck free, head forward and up, back lengthening." Or, he may have reached a point where all he needs to say mentally is the word "lengthening."

The emotional and mental response to the stressful situation is similarly affected. The stress denied to the body is denied to the whole person. As the shoulders are relieved of stress, the whole person is freed of the stressful reaction.

"Wait a minute," you say. "Changing the body will not change the emotions. Don't you have to deal with attitudes and emotions before the body will change?"

Not necessarily so. When people are in some method of psychotherapy, there appears to be a limit to the effects of the therapy as long as there are fixed "sets" to the body. Wilhelm Reich talked of "muscular armoring," and of dissolving it with his type of therapy. The Alexander Technique reaches areas that are not reached in therapy, including Reichian therapy.

The reverse is also true. Progress in Alexander lessons is often limited to some extent if a student has not worked on attitudes and emotional states.

With or without psychotherapy, the Alexander Technique is a pleasurable way to become freer, more open and more aware.

Give yourself directions. At first the changes may be too subtle to notice. But then the joy arrives, ripples at first, then tidal waves.

"Let the neck be free, to let the head go forward and up, to let the back lengthen and widen."

Chapter **8**

Applying the Language of Good Use

LEARNING THE LANGUAGE of good use is like learning a foreign language. At first it seems strange to say things in a different way than you are used to, and you are unsure of yourself; you need to constantly translate from your own language to the new language. When your learning of a foreign language is based on grammar and written exercises, your learning is limited and does not become natural. When you learn grammar *and* are exposed to hearing the language, the language sooner or later becomes second nature; instead of translating from your own language you are *thinking* in the new language and it has become an integral part of you.

The Alexander Technique is a combination of the grammar *and* the exposure to the new language. The grammar of The Alexander Technique is the aspect of learning the more advantageous positions for certain movements, for example, lowering your chin slightly for neck release, bending the knees for bending down and squatting, and various others that I will show you in this chapter. At the same time, with the assistance of the teacher's hands, you are being exposed to what it feels like, and gradually your body learns the new language and you no longer need to consciously direct yourself—it becomes part of your nature.

Relearning a language is faster than learning one that is totally new. As you relearn, there is a familiarity that rings a bell in the mind, and you almost instantly retain the learning that has a familiarity to it. The more recently you had learned—and forgotten—the language, the faster it is relearned.

The Alexander Technique is Relearning the Language of Good Use

We moved well at one time. With some of us, the unlearning of good use started at a very early age, perhaps three years old or five years old, or even earlier. With others, it may not have started until puberty, or late teens, and with others the interference to good use came at a later stage in life.

Although it may seem to some of you that some months of lessons is a long time, it is a very short period of time compared to the many years of misuse. Two half-hour lessons per week for three months would come to a total of twelve to fourteen hours, and over a period of six months would come to approximately thirty hours. From fourteen to thirty hours to unlearn the habits of fifty years! Or the habits of twenty years! Thirty hours to recapture a youthfulness and bouyancy and ease that is fluent and natural! It would take far longer than thirty hours to learn a language, and it would take a minimum of one year of intensive study, homework and practice to become fluent in it.

The role of the Alexander teacher becomes more appreciated as you continue to give yourself directions. On your own, you may be moving from bad use to not-so-bad use, learning the grammar without the fluency that comes from being exposed to the language.

The Alexander teacher is trained to know good use and to help you attain it. With the Alexander teacher, you go from bad to good, not from bad to not-so-bad. You become fluent.

The Alexander teacher observes and senses the subtlest change in the student's body and gives feedback to the student. Sometimes a change is an improvement over the old habit, but is still not fluent good use. The teacher knows the difference. You will definitely benefit from giving yourself directions, but do realize that you will not have changes that are as deep and as subtle as those you get together with the skill of an Alexander teacher.

As a student continues to take lessons he begins to move differently in every activity. This is only the beginning. The process needs to be reinforced. The first changes need to be consolidated and feel natural to permit more subtle improvement.

The more reinforcement there is the greater degree of good use will result. As the reinforcement becomes secure, there is less and less chance that some stressful period can cause a relapse. It is like peeling an onion. Layer after layer of unwanted habits are uncovered and peeled away, habits that could eventually lead to aches and pains that would limit the joy and pleasure of living.

There comes a time when the student and the teacher feel that an excellent level of good use has been reached and is being maintained. We usually agree then that lessons may be discontinued. Some students will want to continue. That may come only once a week or once every two weeks, to feel a "lift" that they are reluctant to give up. Many Alexander teachers have "regulars."

An example is Mitchell Brower, film producer, who came to me for lessons for a few years. He first came because of a painful shoulder, and his realization that poor posture contributed to it. He had been to chiropractors and other physical therapists and would get temporary relief. When he heard of the Alexander Technique, he thought it might help.

Mitchell's shoulder pain disappeared and his posture improved. He had refused my request to take a photograph at his first lesson. Now he regrets it because he would like to be able to show others what a change the Alexander lessons brought him. Many people have remarked on his good posture and do not believe his story of once having been approximately one inch shorter in height, and very slumped with rounded shoulders.

His three-times-a-week Alexander schedule dropped to one visit a week. He maintained his weekly lesson for a few years, for as he puts it, "The Alexander lessons saved my sanity." The world of film producing is one of the most stressful vocations to choose. Alexander lessons are this producer's answer. Mitchell became regarded as being cool and calm in the heat of Hollywood tempests.

Stress and Sanity

How could a technique successful in alleviating a shoulder pain also "save my sanity?"

Well, let's say a movie director called David is on the set and the day's shooting is about to begin. The cast is assembled after hours of costuming and make-up. They are waiting for the leading lady. Then he is told that the leading lady has gone home ill.

He sees red! He sees a filming schedule going down the drain. He sees thousands of dollars in stockholder's money wasted. He sees losses staring him in the face instead of profits, with loss of prestige, and maybe loss of a job.

Look at David. His face is flushed. His fists are clenched. His shoulders have scrunched upwards. His back has collapsed in despair. His mouth is compressed to contain the four-letter words he would like to shout. There is an arch in his back that was not there a moment ago. His legs have become tight from holding back his anger. The back of his neck has tightened and you can see by the way he holds his shoulder that the pain there has increased.

Those around him think: "He looks as if he's going to have a fit." When you add this blow to the others that Michael has been subjected to in the past few days—the script somebody else got, the poor receipts reported on some of his other films, the negative cash flow—David is at the breaking point of his tolerance. Something may have to give and it could be his sanity. He could be risking a nervous breakdown. Certainly, by the "set" of his body he is reinforcing the stress of his anger, impatience, frustration and despair to an intolerable degree.

Now, let's say that David has had Alexander lessons. The news about the leading lady's illness arrives. It is still distressing news, but you would not know it by looking at him. There is no change in his body as he remains lengthened and widened. Should he feel an angry tightening in his body, he recognizes it instantly and automatically releases.

It is as if, through the upward directions, the emotional energy is being released upwards and outwards. It is not suppressed and held in to wreak havoc in the body and in the mind. It is dissipated, as the good direction of the body reinforces expansion and openness.

When the body is maintained free and buoyant, the problems weigh less on the shoulders. They seem "up there" somewhere. With a ton on your shoulders, you cannot be anything but subjective about the stressful circumstances weighing on you. With no weight on your shoulders, you can be objective even in a crisis.

Instead of feeling tempestuous emotions in a crisis, supported by the "invectives" of body language, you go to work constructively to solve the problem. The energy is directed creatively without the short circuits of self-pity, hostility, and attack.

In David's case, the crisis bounces off him. There is even no need for him to give himself Alexander directions. The whole process is automatic, and instantaneous. He sees it as an immunity to stress.

At a recent meeting of the American Association for the Advancement of Tension Control held in Chicago, it was emphasized again and again that tension starts with the brain's issuance of commands to contract muscle groups throughout the body. Athletes who are given tension control training are able to block out crowd noises and squelch butterflies in their stomachs at those crucial moments.

Emotional responses are as evident as physical responses with the Alexander method. A young man came to me for Alexander lessons, looking grim and serious. He told me he was "into meditation" but his face did not look serene. After a few lessons he confessed that he had been accustomed to feeling angry a lot of the time, even when walking down the street. Now he was giving himself Alexander directions and feeling no anger. You could "see" the difference. His face was softer, his personality was warmer.

Physical stress can also be a factor in one's life. It can be a factor, of course, for professionals in spectator sports, but it can also come from the internal environment. One woman with scoliosis, a double

"S" sideways curvature of the spine, came for Alexander lessons. This condition, once it is set at the adult stage, is rarely changeable. The Alexander Technique has been very successful in bringing improvement in this very serious condition, to both adults and children. This lady did see some change—a lessening of the curvature. I will let Dr. Genevieve Meyer describe, in her own words, what the Alexander work has meant to her:

I first started doing Alexander work with Judith Stransky at the beginning of August, 1976, continuing ever since because the benefits and results to me have been constantly remarkable.

At the time I started doing Alexander work I was very worried about the possibility of not being able to continue on with my teaching. At that point in time, I was having great difficulty eating at dinner time, and I felt as if a completely rigid pole was up my spine like a corkscrew. I felt completely twisted and turned around. I could eat okay in the morning; I was having a lot of dizziness during the day, and I had pretty much given up on eating dinner because the strain of standing while cooking and then sitting down to eat was so severe by that time, I could hardly swallow. The physical condition underlying all this is a thoracic and lumbar scoliosis—about a 35 percent curvature. The curvature in the upper back was more pronounced at the time I came to Judith. The right shoulder blade humped out behind so visibly that I would not go anywhere unless I had a sweater on, or a blouse or something thrown over my shoulders. My friends described me as "walking and looking pastorally," like an old woman. The left shoulder, which is now completely normal looking, had begun to turn inwards, and the whole thrust of my body was forward. I also felt as if I had a stomach 3 months or 6 months pregnant.

The first visible effects of the Alexander work were friends noticing that I looked different. Their usual comment was that I must have lost weight. Actually what was happening was that I was standing straighter, without trying to, without effort. I looked younger. Most of all, I began to have hope again.

I would say that physically now, except to the trained observer, I look perfectly normal. If you really know where to look, you can see that the back on the right side is not quite as smooth as on the left. One hip is slightly higher, but I defy anybody to notice that unless I point it out. I feel that I look like a normal human being again, whereas before, I certainly didn't. My body, much of the time, feels much freer and lighter. Before, I used to have a great deal of actual pain, now I would say it's at a level of discomfort and it's intermittent.

These are the obvious physical things, but the psychological turning point for me was after approximately the third lesson. Until then, I was very skeptical and desperate at the same time. I was skeptical because I had tried everything from orthopoedic men, to an osteopath, to acupuncture, and everything was just going downhill. I had emotionally given up; I was restricting my physical activity. I was sitting in recliners all the time and trying to make myself comfortable. My body felt like lead, and my muscles were about as responsive. After about my third Alexander lesson, I began to feel an enormous surge of a need to move physically. The muscles were not strong and couldn't do a lot of walking, or whatever, but I began to feel an energy.

One thing I really want to emphasize for anybody who is not familiar with the Alexander work, who has never tried it, is that it's gradual and you participate in it yourself in the mental sense of giving yourself directions. You give them throughout the day, above and beyond the Alexander lessons. It's not like a massage or a treatment where you go and something gets done to you and then you feel better for a while. It's something in which you, as I've experienced it for myself, are really letting your muscles, your whole body, your spine unlearn all kinds of unnatural ways that we have become used to, and you're going back to what's natural. So, for a while, as in the first three weeks of my Alexander work, my body felt confused. I was used to doing things one way, but I was learning a different way of doing them, and I was practicing the Alexander directions as I would waddle, as I would cook, even as I would try to sit in a chair and read. And, after two to three weeks, things started becoming easier. I remember, in particular, the very dramatic time that an area in my shoulder indicated to me what the directions could do. The shoulder is now totally symptom-free, but since my teen years had given me off and on trouble of a strain in my shoulder and difficulty in turning my head to the right. It was a rainy day and my shoulder was hurting. I had an Alexander lesson scheduled the following morning so that I wasn't overly upset by it, and then I had the sense and happy idea to experiment with it. I tried a whole number of activities, from wiggling my big toe to picking up a pencil off the floor, to getting in and out of the chair, while *not* giving myself directions. And, no matter what I did, whether I was moving that shoulder or not, I would feel the twinge in my shoulder. When I repeated the same actions, *giving myself the directions*, and at this point I was quite new in the work, the shoulder wouldn't hurt. And, that was the thing that really showed me the inner relationships of all the muscles, of the whole body, of the workings of everything, and made a believer out of me, and I use that word very seriously.

From then on, I knew this was the way for me to go, and that improvement was possible. I'm still not at the level that I hope I will eventually reach, but the improvement over the last almost two-year period has been remarkable when I look back. It's a gradual thing—it doesn't happen overnight, and you hit periods where you seem to have plateaus. But, overall, there's much more of a sense of lightness and ease in my body. Where there was constant pain, there is now only intermittent discomfort.

Some of the other things I'd like to say about the Alexander work that are so impressive to me are that you participate in your own recovery. You get a sense of mastery of your own body. You gradually (at least for me) develop a very keen kinesthetic awareness that wouldn't have been possible for me a couple of years ago. I'm aware of sensations, I'm aware of lengthening happening, spontaneously and also when I give myself the directions. It gives me a lot more feedback, so that throughout the day, I can pace myself and move through the day more easily and without strain. And, at times, I really feel good. For me, that's kind of a miracle.

Among the other things that I'd like to say about it is that you can't really explain it to another person. It seems very simple, and yet, it's very, very powerful. You begin to instill in your muscles, or reactivate, the early memories of the muscles, and you don't have to work at it all the time. It works for you without your having to do it.

Just today, when I was at the hairdresser, he commented that I was moving so freely and easily that, to look at me, you wouldn't suspect that I had a back problem. That's where I'm at today, as far as people seeing me. I know that I forget about it for long periods of time. That, also, is so unlike where I was a couple of years ago. I have hopes for even more improvement in the future. I don't know where I would have been without the Alexander work. I hate to even imagine what my life might have been like. At the time that I came to Judith, I saw myself becoming a cripple in a wheelchair. As it is today, I'm functioning well. I'm an associate professor at Cal-State University, Los Angeles. I also run my home. I'm able to do all the watering in the garden, which I had thought I would have to give up forever. I have two volunteer programs working with Senior Citizens. I go out a lot. I eat out a lot. I never thought I could eat dinner out again and really enjoy it. And, now I'm able to do that. I could add more to the list. And, what can I say, except that for me, it's just been sensational. Thank you.

➡ A Bending Change for the Better

Bending is a common movement. You bend to wash your hands, look into a mirror, open a drawer; to pick up an object, take out the garbage, lift a child, shovel snow, get into a car, or pet the dog.

I would like you to see how you bend down. Put the book down, stand up and bend down to pick an imaginary pin off the floor. As you get there, be aware of what you are doing, feeling it in the legs, knees, buttocks, back, neck, head. Are your legs straight or bent?

Do you stick your butt out into the space behind you? What about your neck? Did you tighten and shorten it? And your head? Is it pulled backwards?

Stand up and go near a mirror so that you will be able to see your profile when you bend. Bend again and pick up the pin and then turn your head to look in the mirror and examine the mirror image of yourself.

Some people keep the knees locked when they bend, and their legs close together. This is quite a strain on the lower back. If you did this, spread your feet apart, bend down again, and let your knees and your hip joints bend. See if this is not easier for you. It is almost a semi-squat.

Some people, though they bend their knees and hip joints, *try* to keep their back straight while bending. This makes the buttocks stick out behind and the lower back tighten and arch. It also makes the back of the neck tighter, pulling the head backwards and downwards. And it often forces both heels to lift off the floor, forcing both feet onto the toes while bending, giving an unstable balance. And while they are doing all this, they *feel* straight. They need the mirror to show them the truth.

Let me see if I can help you with my words, since I am not there to help you with my hands. Read this through first and then follow the directions, or have somebody read this to you.

Place a book on the floor in front of your feet. Stand with your knees and feet apart. It is easier to bend this way. Your arms hang loosely at your sides. You look down and see the book on the floor and you wish to pick it up. You make a decision that you will pick it up. With this decision made, *forget about the book*. Do *not* think about it any more.

Instead, *think of your head*. Gently lower your chin slightly, which brings your head slightly forward. *Think* of your head going upwards in small gentle movements. Gradually allow your knees and hip joints to bend, consistently thinking of your head going upwards. As your knees bend, begin to lean forward, continuing to lower your chin and to think of your head going upwards in gentle movements. As you lean forward, you are also bending at your hip joints. Continue bending your knees, leaving your heels on the floor. If you find

BENDING

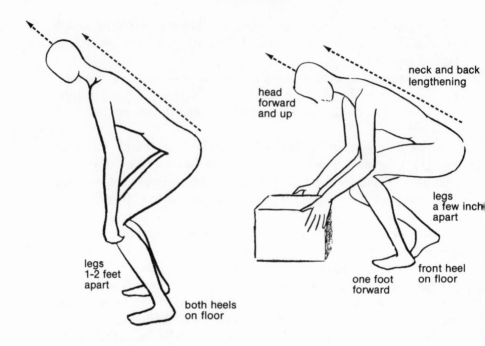

head forward and up

neck and back lengthening

legs a few inch apart

front heel on floor

one foot forward

legs 1-2 feet apart

both heels on floor

GOOD USE

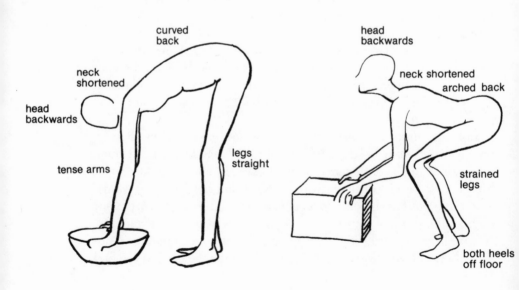

curved back

neck shortened

head backwards

tense arms

legs straight

head backwards

neck shortened

arched back

strained legs

both heels off floor

POOR USE

that you reach a point where your heels want to come up off the floor, then bend further forward with your head and torso. You will find that you will be bending more at the hip joints instead of lifting your heels off the floor.

(A variation of bending is when your feet are only a few inches apart, and you stand with one foot further forward than the other; then, as you bend, your back heel will lift off the floor, while your front heel stays on the floor. This variation is not good for picking up heavy objects.)

Continue bending your knees slowly. This is what is going to get you close to the floor. Do not think about the book. Use your mind to direct your neck to be free, your head to go forward and up, and your back to lengthen. When you are halfway there, your head is no longer going up in the direction of the ceiling, and you need to tell your head to go towards the wall in front of you, "head forward and *out.*" As you continue bending your knees, you arrive closer to the book. Your hands are now very close to the book. Allow one or both hands to gently take the book. *Only your hand moves.* You do not need to tighten your neck or hunch your shoulders. Nothing need happen with your butt or back. You simply put your hand around the book.

Wait. *Do not think of coming up to standing.* Instead, we are going to reverse the process we used for bending, as if we are playing a movie backwards. Allow your legs to unbend, by allowing your knees and hip joints to unbend. In this way, your legs gently straighten. While you allow this, say: "My neck is free; my head is going forward and up; my back is lengthening," or, simply, "lengthening." Once your legs are straight, you are standing up. Do *not* lock your knees. *There is nothing more to do.*

There may be an inclination to do something more with your back and/or legs, in order to get the feeling that you are standing up straight. If you give in to this urge, you will "blow it." You will be overworking. You will be tightening your lower back, legs and neck, and possibly your shoulders. *Instead*, think again of lengthening upwards, toward the ceiling.

Apply this process when bending to open a drawer, to pick up a telephone or any other time that you want to reach down. Instead of

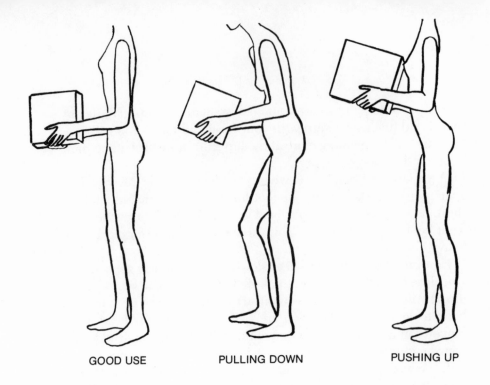

GOOD USE   PULLING DOWN   PUSHING UP

reaching down, think "head forward and up" and "back lengthening," and allow your knees to bend as you allow your head and torso to lean forward. Bend as far as you need to until *it is easy* to reach the object with your hands. *Avoid reaching out or reaching down* with your arms. Let your legs do the movement of bringing you close enough that your hands can *float* towards the object. Then you allow yourself to *unbend gently* and *float upward to standing.*

You may like to repeat this in front of the mirror, using the book. First do it without mental directions, sneaking a sideways peek at your profile before you start and then again when you arrive near the book on the floor, and again when you are standing up. Then bend down again, while giving yourself the mental directions. Look gently to the side at the mirror *only* when you are ready to pick up the book and again when you are standing. You might also like to stop for a moment halfway down and look at yourself. When you go down with

BENDING

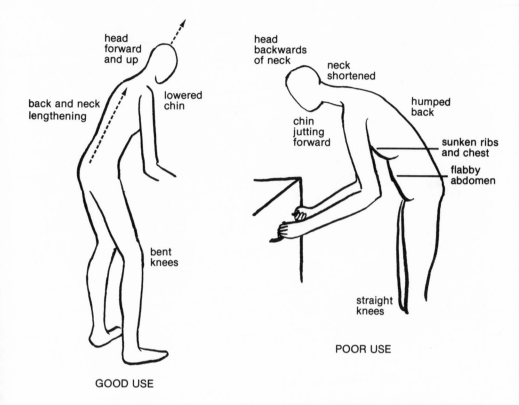

GOOD USE

head forward and up

back and neck lengthening

lowered chin

bent knees

POOR USE

head backwards of neck

neck shortened

humped back

chin jutting forward

sunken ribs and chest

flabby abdomen

straight knees

ease with your mental directions, and without "aiming" to pick up the book, your back is probably straighter than you feel it is, certainly straighter than when you bend down thinking only of picking up the book and not of *how* you move.

Try it also with other objects: picking up a chair, picking up the telephone, opening a drawer, and anything else you wish to do.

Most important of all is that you *feel easier, smoother and lighter* when you bend with good use.

At first, you may feel that your back is not straight—let your mirror show you whether it is or not. Eventually, you will come to know when your back is straight without the mirror.

Regardless of whether your back feels "straight" to you or not, you will have a feeling of *ease*—and that is good use, that is the Alexander Technique.

When you have sensed this ease in bending down and know how

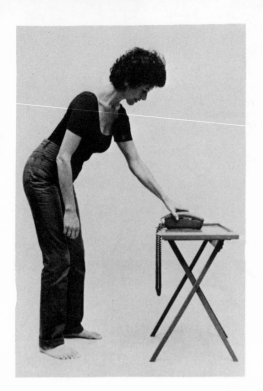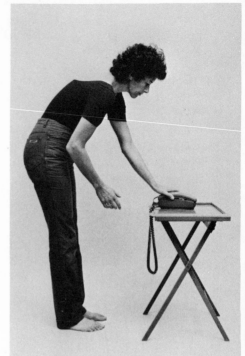

to recapture it, use it for picking up a heavier object, such as a chair. *The weight of the chair will vary according to your use.* When you use too much tension in your body, the chair will be heavier. When you use good direction in your body, the chair will be light.

Try it, and find out for yourself.

➡ How to Lengthen While Moving

Moving slowly is necessary *while learning.* This gives you time to give your directions all the way, and also allows you the opportunity to sense when you are "contracting," or tightening. When you move fast you do not notice when you have started to contract and therefore do not have a chance to release into length.

In daily life, moving unnaturally slowly is not recommended. Move normally, and *take a split second before starting a movement to direct yourself, instead of rushing into the movement. Avoid rushing.* Move at a pace that is normal, neither at a snail's pace, nor rushing as if you have a train to catch. You may repeat your directions *while* doing a movement, whether it be bending, sitting, standing or whatever.

Waiting for a split second before doing a movement to say "head forward and up" or "lengthening" will be very rewarding. I recommend that you give your directions, *"before, during and after."*

This helps you to have the experience of one movement flowing into another, as if they are all one. All movement is "lengthening," and being still is also "lengthening"—it is all the same.

➡ What is Lengthening?

"Lengthening" is the normal state of your muscles.

"Contraction" is an abnormal state.

This is what these two words indicate in our Alexander "language." When technically describing how muscles function, this is not quite accurate.

To be extremely accurate, the word contraction applies to a normal condition of the muscles, just as the word tension does; contraction is the same as tension. To make it clear: there is a certain degree of tension, or contraction, required in muscles in order for you to be standing up or sitting up. If all muscles were loose and floppy, you would be in a heap on the floor, or on the chair. There is an additional degree of tension, or contraction, required to move muscles, and this is normal. When certain muscles contract to move, the opposite muscles lengthen; for example, when you bend your arm, the muscles on the inside of your arm contract or shorten, and the muscles on the outside extend or lengthen. Without that, you would not be able to bend your arm. *The normal degree of tension, or contraction, feels effortless.* A normal degree of contraction is required in good use.

OVER-CONTRACTION, or OVER-TENSION IS THE CULPRIT OF MISUSE.

Most of us are over-contracting, both while standing up and while sitting up, and while moving from one position to another. We experience this as "tense muscles," or a "tense body." When we over-contract constantly, those muscles remain contracted or shortened and are unable to achieve their full length again on their own.

You see this in elderly people who are bent over and cannot straighten up; even their elbows are permanently bent. Many of us have over-contracted muscles to a lesser degree, and as we continue misusing them, they become more and more contracted, or shortened. Over-contracting means over-working certain muscles, and the opposite muscles are under-working. The over-worked muscles are tight, and the under-worked muscles are flabby.

Alexandrians use the word "lengthening" to request the over-contracted muscles to release from their contracted state to a normal state, as a normal muscle is longer than a short or tight muscle. The word "lengthen" encourages the release of the excessive contraction. We popularly use the terms "lengthen" and "contract," just as in daily life you popularly use the word "tension" when what you really mean is "over-tense," or "excessive tension." "Lengthening" is Alexandrian shorthand for "normal state of the muscles," and "contraction" is our shorthand for "over-worked and over-tense muscles."

➡ Take Inches Off Your Waist
With Lengthening and Widening

Many people ask what I mean by "widening." Some of them are concerned that they are going to get fatter. There is no need to fear.

Widening is the same as lengthening, only it is applied to the muscles that go *across the torso*, in the front and in the back, while lengthening is applying to the muscles that go up and down the torso. Muscles that go across the torso, either laterally or diagonally, contract at the same time as muscles that go up and down the torso. When the "up-and-down" muscles in the front of your torso over-contract so do the muscles that go "across" the front of your torso, and the same happens when the back muscles contract. This brings about a narrowing, as seen in narrow shoulders, a small chest, tight ribs, sway back. When the excessive contraction of the "across" muscles is released, your shoulders and chest become broader and your sway back vanishes. Result: broader chest and narrower waist.

The "across" muscles cannot release into length by themselves, it happens simultaneously with the releasing into length of the "up-

and-down" muscles, and the whole effect is a longer, smoother body, with longer, smoother muscles, broader shoulders, uplift in the bosom, broader chest, smaller waist, smaller hips, and longer, straighter legs.

➡ The Uplift That Can Be Yours

"Take Inches Off Your Waist," or "Exercise Without Exercises" was the title of the feature article in the fashion magazine *Harper's Bazaar*, April 1967. This article was about the Alexander Technique, written by Edward Maisel, Director of the American Physical Fitness Research Institute. This article is reproduced by some of the Alexander Centers listed in the Appendix, and available to the public.

The lengthening and widening of the Alexander Technique is an effortless, pleasurable way to improve your figure, for both men and women. Many report a loss of inches in waist and hips, even without a loss of weight, and this comes together with an increase in height, smoother stomach, broader chest and a fuller bosom. Some students find that even when they gain a few pounds, their clothes do not become tight because of the renewed elongation and slenderness in their torso. And many students of either sex find that they need to take a smaller size in their pants and their belts, and women students often need to buy bras one size larger.

Here is the story of an 81-year-old lady who came for lessons. She was referred to me because she had not recovered well from a broken hip. Her walk was feeble, she limped, used a cane, and she was becoming more and more limited in her activities. She was always dressed in black, which contrasted with her white hair. Her Vermont background gave her a dignity which demanded respect and admiration.

After several lessons, she was walking freely and energetically, barely using the cane, and had great relief from the residual pain of the hip operation. When she came in for her seventh lesson, Mary's usually serious face was wreathed in smiles.

"Judith," she said, "would you believe this at my age: I am getting an uplift! When I undress, I find my bosom has an uplift to it that I have not seen for years and years."

Uplift is where you find it. The Alexander Technique is an uplift. Lengthening and widening is an uplift.

➡ Shoulder Embrace
Hug Yourself for Widening and Lengthening

Now I would like to share with you an exercise that will help to release your upper back. In addition to improving the lengthening and lightening of your body, it will also help you to experience widening across your shoulders, and across your upper back.

Lie down on the floor, bend your knees, and spread your legs apart and your feet apart, moving one leg at a time. Take your right arm, lift it over your chest and put your right hand under your left armpit so that the fingers of your right hand touch your left shoulder blade. Now take your left arm and move it over your chest and right arm and bring the fingers of your left hand to touch your right shoulder blade. *Very gently* roll your chest right and left while your

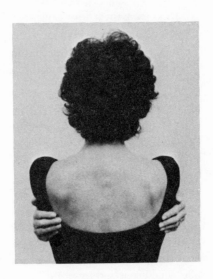

fingers are touching your shoulder blades. You are embracing yourself and hugging yourself as you tilt your chest right and left. Do not tilt your knees. In order to get more effect on the upper back, you need to keep the knees still. Let your knees continue to point up to

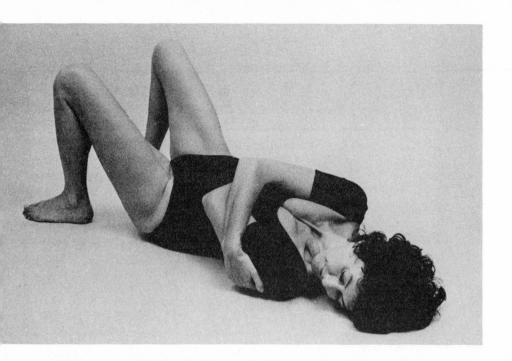

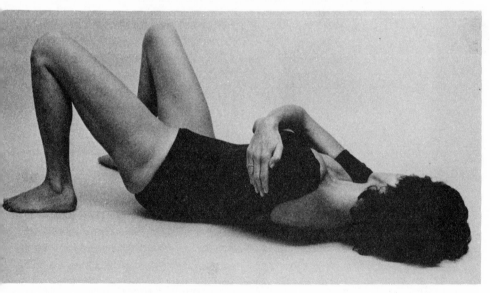

the ceiling and let *only your upper torso move*, rolling right and left. It is a rolling movement, and your upper back is curved when you hold your shoulder blades like this with your hands. Allow your head and eyes to roll with your chest.

All the time, *think that you are loving yourself*. When you love yourself, your muscles relax, the tension releases, they become softer and smoother. Think of how you relax when someone else loves you, and embraces you lovingly; you can do it for yourself.

After a few movements, come to the middle and slowly change over the crossing of your arms, and roll again right and left. This time, when you tilt your chest to the right, let your head and eyes roll to the left; when you tilt your chest to the left, let your head and eyes roll to the right. Your head and eyes are going opposite to your chest. As you do this, you will find that there is a corkscrew movement in your upper spine. This is very helpful for undoing tension in the neck and upper back. It is necessary, though, to *do it softly and gently*. Now do it a little bit faster and a little more playfully.

After you have done it this way a few times, allow your head and eyes to go in the same direction as your chest again, and continue to do the movement softly, a little fast and playfully. After a few more times, come to resting in the middle; very gently bring your arms down alongside your body and gently lower your legs one at a time.

See how your back feels as it lies on the floor, and also your head. I think you will find there is some change in your whole back; now think of your shoulder blades and you may find there is an even greater change there. Do they feel as if they are more spread out across the floor, lying more smoothly and more evenly? Notice your chest. Is there more space in your chest, as if the front part of your upper torso has also widened and created more space inside? How is your breathing? I think you will find there is a change in your breathing. Please do not try to change it, simply notice it and see whether it is different than before. Is it smoother, easier, deeper?

Slowly bend your knees one at a time, roll over onto one side, gently roll onto your hands and knees, and come up to standing. Walk around and see whether you feel changes in your body as you walk. Walk normally, do not try to change your walk. Breath normally. You may find that what is normal now, is rather different than what was normal before you did this exercise.

After the shoulder embrace, you could be experiencing what we call "widening" in the Alexander Technique, as well as what we call "lengthening." The lengthening would be felt as feeling taller and lighter, the widening would be felt across your shoulders, upper

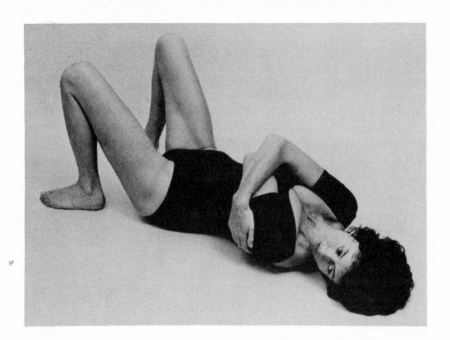

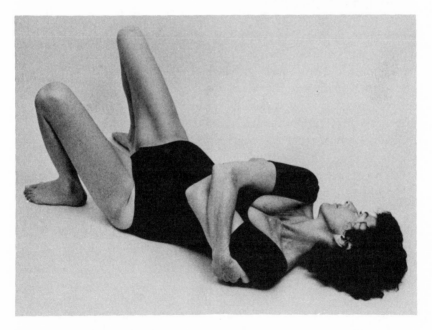

back, and chest. You may feel there is more space inside you, that your shoulders are spread further apart from each other, that your chest is wider, and that there is more space across your upper back;

this would feel light and easy, expanding outwards into space and upwards into space.

➤ Washing Your Hands of Misery

If I could be as successful in getting you to bend well via this book as Alexander teachers are in an Alexander lesson, you would be on the threshold of a new life.

It is a life where your body is no longer a burden to itself and a distraction to your mind. A lighter body and a more tranquil mind spell joy. It is the joy of an easier life, mentally and physically.

I have taken you through the basic movements of the Alexander lessons, the basic movements of your life. I cannot think "neck free" for you. *You* need to think it. This is true in the Alexander lesson, also. I can only remind the student to give himself directions. I cannot think the thoughts for him.

Every motion you make with your body will be affected as you apply your mental directions. Take washing your hands.

Misuse of your body while washing your hands may appear to be a trivial matter. Your hands are washed properly whether or not your back, neck and shoulders are held properly. Still, it reinforces misuse in other movements and contributes to the sapping of energy, the distortion of the body, and the distraction of the mind.

Would you like to wash your hands now? You may be washing your hands of more than you think. Coupled with Alexander directions for other basic movements you may be washing your hands of a lot more discomfort than dust and grime.

How do you usually wash your hands? Go to a sink. Turn on the faucet. Pick up the soap. Wash your hands. Be aware of your neck, shoulders, back, and knees. Before you dry your hands, remember whether you locked your knees, how you bent down, and whether there was tightening in your neck or shoulders.

Now prepare to wash your hands a second time, with mental directions, Alexander style. Take a moment to decide to wash your hands. Decide that you are going to turn on the faucet, pick up the soap and wash your hands. Now remove all thoughts of washing your hands from your mind and substitute mental directions. You will be directing your body to accomplish your decision in the easiest possible way, without thinking of the goal.

WASHING AT THE SINK

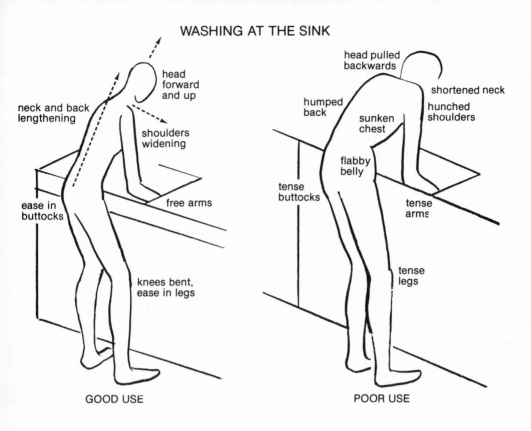

GOOD USE — head forward and up; neck and back lengthening; shoulders widening; ease in buttocks; free arms; knees bent, ease in legs

POOR USE — head pulled backwards; shortened neck; hunched shoulders; humped back; sunken chest; flabby belly; tense arms; tense buttocks; tense legs

Stand in front of the sink with your legs slightly apart. Lower your chin slightly and allow your knees to bend gently, turn on the water, take the soap gently, and wash your hands.

When you are finished, instead of thinking about coming up to dry your hands, gently allow your legs to unbend and straighten, as well as your hip joints. You undo the leg movement that brought you into bending, instead of thinking of straightening up. Coming up out of a bend is simply *undoing* what brought you into a bend. Thinking of it this way is much easier on you than thinking of straightening up.

This is a slighter motion than picking up an object from the floor. Good use is essential, whether a movement is large or small, frequent or infrequent. Good use leads to more good use.

▶ Writing at a Desk

One of the most common occupations at home or at work is writing. Desk workers, whether they be students, housewives who write letters at home, or office workers who type or write reports, frequently develop poor writing habits.

If you were to scan the usual scene at an office, you would see one person writing with a shoulder hunched up, another with both shoulders scrunched together, another might be twisting the body to the side. Still others slump down, lean over, or stiffen up. Other less obvious bad habits would also be present, such as a stiff neck, unnecessary pressure in the fingers and rigidity of the wrists.

Frequently, without my working with an Alexander student directly at the desk, an improvement will occur. As a result the writing flows and becomes easier. College students find that their papers and report writing become more fluent.

Many people who sit at a typewriter for hours complain of an aching back or weary shoulders. With the Alexander Technique, both the obvious and the subtle postural and muscular misuses melt away and with them go the energy drain, pains and aches.

When writing is done by hand, it bears evidence of a person's feelings and attitudes. Handwriting experts produce a great deal of accurate information about the writer's personality and state of mind from his writing.

We develop handwriting habits that derive from our mind-body partnerships. Change one of the partners, or both, and the handwriting changes. Graphotherapy teaches a change in handwriting which results in corresponding changes in the personality. Writing is a neuromuscular activity. Change one part and you affect the other. This is merely another manifestation of the many parts that go to make up the jigsaw puzzle.

Alexander teachers do not attempt to change handwriting. But when they work with an Alexander student, the handwriting often will change.

It can be minor, perhaps coming out of a changed position of arm and paper. Or, the change can be considerable, as the writer himself changes from a bitter, pained individual to a joyous person, freed from the imprisonment from which he was suffering.

Observe yourself at a desk, while writing, and see if you can sense whether you are leaning or twisting to one side, whether your head is pulled downwards to one side and your legs entangled and tense.

You can help yourself by sitting on the chair with good direction, and with both feet on the floor in front of you, as you did when learning to sit in preparation for standing up. With slightly lowered chin, and upward mental directions, allow your forehead and torso to lean forward gently as if you are coming up to standing, and let your hands move lightly into place on the desk and allow yourself to write. You may find that you cannot maintain this easy centered condition of your body because the paper is at an angle which forces you to twist around. Change the angle of the paper.

Check yourself in front of a mirror. If you have a light, portable mirror you could prop it up against a wall in front of your desk to see yourself in it and see whether you are centered. If you are not, stop writing and think of sitting on your chair with good direction, and then observe yourself in the mirror as you start to lean forward gently, thinking upwards, to begin writing. You would be able to see in the mirror if you start to lean to one side with either your head, shoulders, torso or hips. You could add a very useful direction: "Head forward and up *and centered*" in addition to "neck free" and "back lengthening and widening."

You could help yourself further by re-experiencing sitting at a desk with the mirror at your side, showing you your profile as you sit and lean forward to write.

A lightweight, portable, inexpensive door mirror, usually found at Woolworth's and Newberry's, would be a good investment. It is easier to move a portable mirror than to move a desk close to a mirror.

You can help yourself with your writing in another simple way. Every now and again, allow yourself to come to standing—with Alexander direction, naturally—and take a walk around the room or do something different, then resume your writing. This will relieve accumulating tension in your body.

▶ Sitting at the Typewriter

In addition to sitting at the typewriter with your newfound awareness and Alexander directions, there are certain technical changes that are often required to improve our level of ease.

Have your typewriter on a typing table, or any other table that is approximately the same height as the typewriter table. You will notice that typewriter tables are not as high as standard tables or desks. If the table is not low enough, then sit on one or two cushions. To prevent strain and tiredness in your hands, arms, and shoulders, and in your neck and back, your hands and forearms should be on a plane that is parallel to the floor, and not at an upward angle from your elbows. I have sometimes typed at my dining table, and I sat on two firm cushions to bring myself high enough so that I could have my arms in this position while typing. Sit with your feet on the floor, and legs and feet comfortably apart.

When copying from material, do not have the pages you are copying from lying flat on the table. This brings strain into the neck. Get a stand from a stationer's store, so that the pages can be upright. These stands are very simple and inexpensive, and are usually called typing stands. If that is not available, ask for a book stand, which is a similar type of stand and will serve the same purpose. Many people who type have relieved themselves of neck pains by using a stand.

▶ Court Reporting

Here is the story of how I helped a court reporter relieve pain in her upper back by changing some of her working conditions.

This lovely young woman came for lessons for two reasons: first, she had read about the Alexander Technique and wanted the general improvement it offered; second, she had a pain in her upper back near her shoulder blade which had become quite severe since she had been transferred to criminal court, where there was an overload of work and stress.

Each time she had a lesson, she felt marvelous and her pain disappeared. She often arrived feeling very tired, exhausted in body and mind, and would leave feeling light, buoyant and energetic, and ready to continue her transcription work at home. However, her pain would recur between lessons. After two or three weeks, I asked her how she worked at her steno machine in court. She explained that the machine sat on a small table, and because she wore skirts to court (in that particular court women were not allowed to wear pants at that time), she sat with her legs to one side of the table; it was to the left. I asked if she would be willing to sit straight ahead and spread her legs a little apart. She answered no, that would be too immodest. I suggested, instead, that I meet her in court one day, after work, to see if I could help her. We made a date, and when I was there, she showed me her small table and steno machine, and I watched her as she worked. I observed that, because her legs were twisted to the left, her lower torso was also twisted to the left, while her hands, arms, shoulders, neck and head were facing straight ahead. This brought a twist into her upper back. Also, her table was not at the best height.

I then made some suggestions. I showed her that she could move her chair and her machine slightly to the left of the center of the table; in this way she could have her knees straight ahead with one leg on each side of the left front table leg, without spreading her legs apart. She tried this out and felt quite comfortable with the new conditions. We also adjusted her table to a more appropriate height. She worked easily and well with the changes, and experienced no more pain in her upper back.

➡ Holding a Telephone, Eating and Drinking

The poor habits in common with these activities are that people often *go down to the object instead of bringing the object up to them.*

When eating or drinking, instead of leaning downwards, collapsing your torso and squashing your digestive organs, bring the food, or the drink, to your mouth, letting your hands and arms move lightly upwards.

When, for some reason, you wish to get closer to the food or drink without lifting it far from the table—for example, when your soup is hot—you can get closer to the food by leaning forward, with a lowered chin, and with Alexandrian length (see section on Writing at a Desk, P. 225).

With a telephone, as with eating and drinking, *do not go down to the telephone*, but *bring the telephone up to you.*

Some people hold the telephone with their shoulder while occupying both hands with some other activity, usually writing. Try to always have one hand free to hold the telephone. If your office activities make this impossible, save the wear and tear on your body and get a remote telephone appliance, which you place on your desk instead of holding a telephone to your ear. A less expensive item, although not as effective, is a shoulder support for the telephone; this

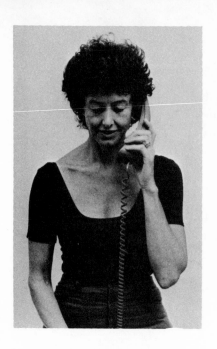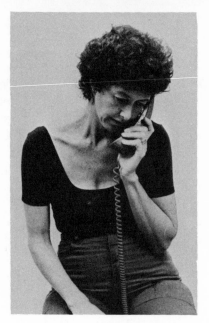

gadget is attached to the ear-and-mouthpiece of the telephone and sits on your shoulder, supporting the telephone close to your ear while you are talking. These are usually available at stationery stores.

Search for ways to make your life comfortable while eating, drinking, talking on the phone, and other everyday activities.

➤ Rest Breaks

A frequent rest break is a very good preventive against mounting tension and aches. This is a very important thing to apply to *any* activity you become involved in that results in your becoming tense and/or suffering from aches or pains.

Many people protest that they do not notice time go by when they are involved in such activities. There is an answer to this. Set an alarm, or timer, to ring after ten minutes, or twenty minutes, to remind you to take a brief break and put a stop to accumulating tension. As you improve the ease of your use, you could extend the time period to half an hour or longer. Remember, prevention is better than cure.

Brief, frequent rest breaks are so effective that you will be able to do more, for a longer period of time, and without the pain of accumulated stress in your body.

➡ Sleeping Positions—Good and Bad

Misuse of body can occur while you are asleep as well as awake. You may think that such misuse is not under your conscious control, instead, you should realize that *poor* sleep habits are acquired and you can acquire *good* sleep habits in their place.

What is good use in sleeping for one person may not be appropriate for another. The first sleep position I recommend is not ideal for everyone, and I will recommend others.

The position is lying on your stomach, *with one knee bent*, and the head turned to one side, *without a pillow*. Try it, according to the following directions.

Lie on the floor on your stomach, with your left ear on the floor and legs apart. Gently slide your right knee up the floor towards your head, bending it until it is at approximately a 90-degree angle. Bending one leg like this relieves tension in your lower back. It would be harmful to your lower back to lie on your stomach with both legs straight, therefore *bending one knee is essential*. A comfortable position for your arms is to let your right arm lie on the floor in front of your face, with the elbow bent at a right angle, and palm down; your left arm lies on the floor alongside your body, palm up. This allows your shoulders to lie freely.

To turn to the other side: gently straighten your right leg, slowly turn your head to the other side gently draw up your left knee. Straighten your right arm down the floor and bend your left arm. You may sleep on either side.

What I like about this sleeping position is that it allows the whole back and spine to be lengthened and allows the shoulders to be free.

SLEEP POSITION

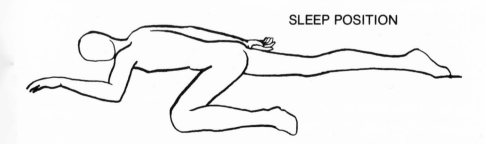

It is important *not to use a pillow in this position*, as that would push your head backwards and tighten your neck on one side, and you could wake up with a pain in your neck and one shoulder.

The movement of changing from one side to the other is a very pleasurable relaxation movement which you could do for yourself at any time; if you are a person who does a routine set of exercises, you could include this as a warmup and muscle-relaxant.

Some women do not like this sleeping position because, as they put it, "it squashes my bosom." Only large-bosomed ladies have this complaint. I suggest that they put a small or medium pillow under the midriff. This relieves the pressure of the bed on their bosom. If a large pillow is used under the midriff because of a correspondingly large bosom, then a small pillow under the head will also be necessary.

Pregnant women will find this a particularly relaxing position. As they become larger in the last months of pregnancy, they will need to put a pillow under the knee that is bent.

Try out this sleeping position tonight. Anything new is less accommodating; what you need to do is persist night after night and try and fall asleep in this position. If the new position is so unfamiliar that it keeps you awake, use your familiar position to go to sleep. One night you will fall asleep in your new position and wake up more relaxed than before, and you will have gained a new habit that will enhance your nightly rest.

Those with neck pains usually cannot use this position as keeping the head turned to one side is too painful. It would defeat our purpose if you could not get a good night's sleep.

Sleep is very important for our well-being. Your muscles and body cannot move lightly and easily during the day when you do not have enough sleep. Muscles lose their elasticity when they are not getting an adequate amount of rest. So be sure that you get enough sleep every night to maintain the fluency of your body.

For those who have neck pain problems, the position I recommend is: lie on your side with your knees drawn up in front of you, one leg on top of the other. Your arms are in front of you, one on top of the other, elbows bent, palms touching each other. Here you do need a pillow, usually two, preferably firm ones. If your pillows are

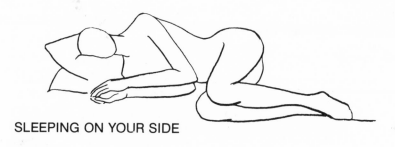

SLEEPING ON YOUR SIDE

not firm, or are very flat, you may even need three. The way to determine the number of pillows you need under your head is to see when your neck is able to go straight out. The pillow height should be enough to maintain your neck in an uninclined, straight-out position. A neck pushed into a curve to one side or the other is not a "happy" neck. "Straight-out" your neck is free and lengthened.

Lying with knees bent, the back is free to lengthen. You may choose to have only one knee bent, then it should be the upper leg that is bent.

In special instances, such as after an operation, a person can lie only on the back. Any other position can be painful. In these cases, I recommend that while lying on your back, you use one or two pillows under your head and also pillows under your knees. Propping up your head and knees with pillows helps to release the back tension. On your back you need less pillow height under your neck than when lying on your side, just enough to allow the neck and head to be going outwards. This is usually one or two pillows. Use enough pillow height under the knees to maintain them about one-third bent or half bent.

SLEEPING ON YOUR BACK

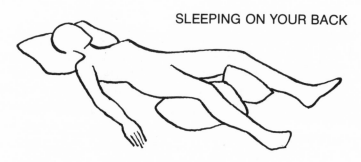

For further information on sleeping positions, and what they indicate about your personality, I recommend *Sleep Positions—The Night Language of the Body* by Samuel Dunkell, M.D.* This book reveals your personality through your sleep position, and helps develop the awareness we need about our sleep positions. This awareness, as in our waking movements and positions, is a necessary step to changes for the better. Again, change the body, even while asleep, and you change the personality.

A *recommendation for sleep* that I have to offer is to lightly think of your Alexander directions when lying in bed preparing to sleep. Give yourself your directions also when you wake up.

Some of my students have found that their bodies feel different all day when they lie on the floor and direct, as I have described to you on pages 19–2, first thing in the morning after getting out of bed. It takes only a few minutes.

The Alexander lessons induce good directions at all times, and this includes the time one spends sleeping. One of my students had evidence of this. He was a scientist who traveled a good deal to conferences in various parts of the country. He told me one day, "Judith, I now know I have Alexander direction even while I am asleep."

"How do you know that?" I asked, wondering how he knew what went on in his sleep.

"When I travel to and from airports in a taxi, I frequently doze off. On awakening, I find my chin down and my head dropped forward onto my chest. However, on this last trip, I dozed off as usual and when I awoke I found I was sitting fully erect. I now have good direction while asleep."

▶ Carrying a Bag on One Side

Many people are "pulled down" on one side, usually the right side. The right shoulder is lower, and the distance between the armpit and the waist on the right side is shorter than on the left side. Often the right hip is higher than the left one. Observe yourself in the mirror and see which side is "pulled down" in your body.

*Signet, New York, N.Y., 1978.

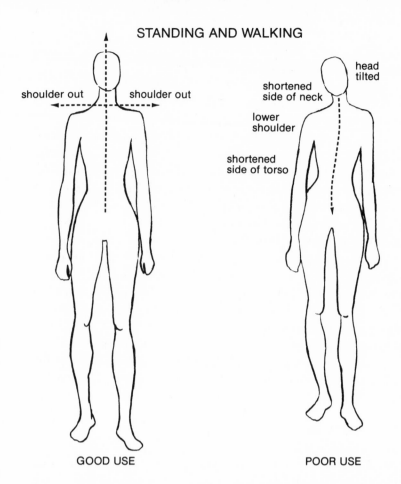

STANDING AND WALKING

shoulder out   shoulder out

head tilted

shortened side of neck

lower shoulder

shortened side of torso

GOOD USE   POOR USE

Regardless of whether it is the right side or the left side, the "pulled down" side is usually the side on which your carry something, either a purse, a shoulder bag, an attaché case, or a suitcase. The extra weight of the object you are carrying pulls you down further and further on that side. This can lead to problems of the spine and back, as both the spine and the back muscles are being pulled out of a good alignment and into a curve, with a corresponding squashing together of the vertebrae and of the muscles in the center of the curve. As many of you have experienced, some back and spinal problems are extremely painful, and often lead to pain in one or both legs.

To prevent and alleviate this is very simple. Do not always carry your bag in the same hand. *Change hands frequently.* You do not need to have equal time on each side, and you do not have to have an alarm clock with you to time each side. Instead, use your awareness. Be aware when the bag is starting to feel heavier, and immediately switch it to the other hand. Each side is different and one side will probably last longer than the other side. Eventually, as your two sides become more equal, the length of time on both sides will become more equal. Ideally, switch hands *before* your arm gets tired, *before* the bag starts to feel heavier.

Naturally, adding your Alexander directions is going to help immeasurably: "Neck free, head forward and up, back lengthening and widening." As the weight of a bag could drag your shoulder down, you can give yourself some additional assistance with the direction "Shoulders out." Give the direction to both shoulders, even if you are carrying a bag in only one hand. "Shoulders out" means that your left shoulder goes towards the left, and your right shoulder goes towards the right. Remember to say "Shoulders out" also when you are carrying a bag in both hands. "Shoulders out" cannot substitute for your basic "lengthening" direction, but add it on whenever you want to. Say your directions silently, lightly and rapidly, and easily.

➡ Carrying a Shoulder Bag

The difficulty with a shoulder bag is that it often feels as if it is going to slip off your shoulder, so you hunch up your shoulder on that side to prevent the strap from slipping down. An easy way to take care of this is to hold the shoulder strap lightly with your hand, near your shoulder. If your shoulder bag is on your right side, use your right hand; on the left side, use your left hand.

If the shoulder bag is heavy, it is pulling you down on that side, and if it is also likely to slip off your shoulder, your shoulder is scrunching up to prevent the strap from slipping. Now you have a double assault of misuse—all because of a shoulder bag. You can easily relieve the weight of the bag by holding the bag from underneath with your hand; use the hand on the same side as the bag.

Each time you carry a shoulder bag, switch it from side to side frequently. And remember the formula for good use: "Neck free, head forward and up, back lengthening and widening and shoulders out"; or use the abbreviated version; "Lengthen, and shoulders out."

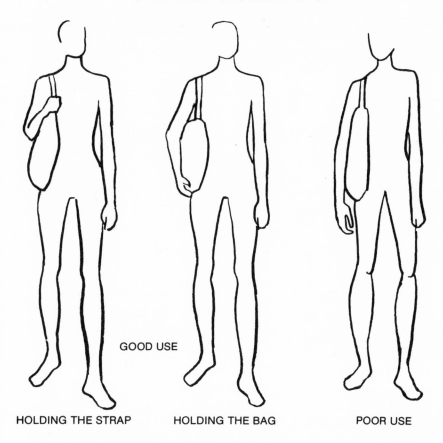

GOOD USE

HOLDING THE STRAP   HOLDING THE BAG   POOR USE

▶ Carrying a Baby

Many mothers have actually caused a curvature in their spine, and a tilted pelvis, by carrying the baby on one side, resting the weight of the baby on the hip on that side. As a result, the hip on that side juts outwards and is higher than the hip on the other side, and this has made the spine curve sideways, which can lead to severe back problems.

Instead, when holding or carrying the baby, *do not jut one hip to the side*, let your hips remain level, and direct your back to go upwards and outwards ("lengthening and widening"), and let your arm support the baby. If your arm is held low enough, you can support it on your hip bone, but *do not bring your hip up to your arm.*

Change sides frequently. Do not always carry the baby on one

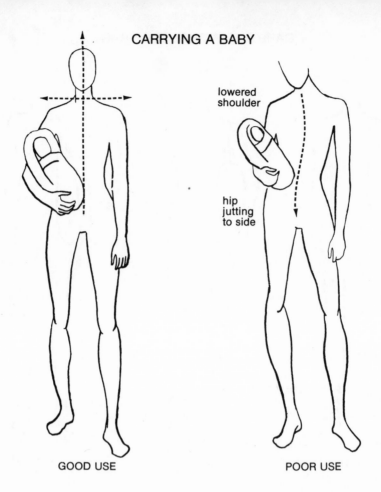

CARRYING A BABY

lowered
shoulder

hip
jutting
to side

GOOD USE   POOR USE

side. You can prevent future back problems by changing the baby often from one side to the other. As you carry your baby, think of lengthening upwards and of *being centered.* Not only will you be preventing future trouble for yourself, you will also have a nice effect on your baby, who will experience being held against an easy, flowing body. Perhaps your baby will get Alexandrian direction by osmosis that will go beyond babyhood. "Neck free, head forward and up, back lengthening and widening."

▶ Lifting Heavy Objects

Avoid lifting, moving, or carrying heavy objects as much as possible. Do not be heroic. Ask someone to help you. If it is something that is not a necessity, don't do it. If it is something that is a necessity, ask for help. If there is no one around to help you, see if

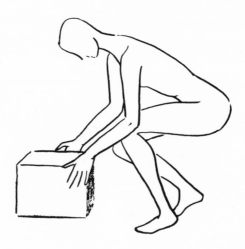

there is some easy way to move that object. If it is a piece of furniture, perhaps you can push it instead of lifting it. Perhaps you can slide it. If so, I would like you to do it in the way that I show you in the drawing above. Do not keep your legs straight. Bend your knees and bend at your hip joints. By bending your knees and hip joints and leaning forward with your head and torso, you could prevent back trouble or going into muscle spasm or straining muscles. When you stop, unbend gently while thinking of "lengthening."

Another way of moving things easily is to put wheels or coasters on them. You can buy wheels for suitcases. There are wheels for furniture and heavy objects that you can put on temporarily, and wheels that you can attach permanently. There are wheels you can buy to place under furniture so that you can wheel it across the floor. Installing glides under furniture allows you to glide the furniture across the floor more easily. Find easy ways to do things instead of the most difficult way.

If there is no way out of picking up or moving a heavy object, use the directions in the sections "A Bending Change for the Better," page 210, and "How to Lengthen While Moving," page 216. Move slowly, in slow motion, move carefully and with Alexander directions. Stop frequently to rest from the burden. In general, take good care of yourself with thoughtfulness, common sense, and awareness.

➡ Jogging and Running

Often people ask me about jogging and running. Some of them are Alexander students and some of them are not. Usually my Alexander students do not have to ask about it, because they have learned through the Alexander Technique how to use themselves well in all activities, including jogging and running.

I am often told by people that when they jog or run, they get muscle cramps in their legs or an aching back, or a stiff neck, their feet hurt, or their heels ache. I show them how to change the way they hold their bodies, and introduce them to the Alexander directions.

When you watch people jogging and running, you will see that many of them throw their shoulders back, throw their chests out in front and throw their heads backwards; the result is a tight neck, a tight back, and extra tension in the arms and legs. You often can see the muscles in the legs straining, and the muscles in the shoulders and arms held rigidly.

Instead of doing that, lean forward *slightly* with your torso, lower your chin slightly and tell your head it is going forwards and upwards and tell your torso that it is lengthening, following the head upwards. Think of the top of your head leading the whole movement, as it goes forwards and upwards. When you lower your chin *do not think* of dropping it downwards, instead *think of going forwards and upwards. Do not push* your head upwards, *do not push* your neck upwards, or try and push your back upwards. Use only mental thoughts: "neck free, head forward and up, back lenghtening and widening."

Because of your lowered chin and leaning forward, you will be looking down, and you could complain that you would bump into things. I recommend that, while leaving your chin slightly lowered and leaning forwards and upwards, you open your eyelids more, so that you can be *looking down in the distance* far ahead of you. Now you will have a vast area of peripheral vision and can see all the things in your vicinity, and ahead of you.

When you give your upward directions, your torso becomes lighter and relieves the pressure on your legs, your legs move more freely with less strain and there is less pressure on the feet and on the heels, and your arms can move freely. Your whole experience of jogging and running will not only be improved in performance, but can also become a joyous experience. Instead of it being the cramped, distorted you, it is the original free, joyous you, having a beautiful experience in jogging and running.

➡ Here And Now

Most of us are preoccupied with the past and with the future. We blame the way we are on past events and feel resentments and hang-ups. We wonder how we are going to arrive at our goal in the future, and experience this as worry and anxiety. Seldom do these dark clouds of the past merging with the dark clouds of the future permit light to enter—the light of the here and now.

Alexander understood that what we do in this instant dictates what will happen in the next. He understood the importance of the present instant. He understood how the effects of the past could be replaced by different mental directions, a term that produces results figuratively and literally. His understanding has led to a body-mind teaching technique which restores the present to the spotlight of human consciousness. Alexander lessons bring the student into the here and now.

We hear a lot about the here and now from "new-age" types. Starting with flower children and continuing with hippie and drug culture types, the here and now was the averred purpose for the life style. But still, the past and future eclipsed the present. Glimpses of joy may have been experienced but were quickly enveloped by new-age complications involving yesterday's carryovers and tomorrow's expectations.

Several years ago, a young Greenwich Village lad, whom I shall call Henry, came to me for lessons. He was heavily into marijuana, although I did not know that at first. His body was slender and very slumped down, with a big sway in his back and very rounded shoulders. His face also sagged. "I want to do this right," he said to me on arrival. "How often should I come?" I suggested three times a week was the best way. He readily agreed.

We began the lesson and I have never seen, before or since, such a rapid and dramatic response. There were enormous changes in one lesson. I had taken photos of him at the beginning of the lesson, which I like to do for my records. Usually I take another series of photos towards the conclusion of a period of lessons. With him, the results were so astounding in thirty minutes that I took another set of pictures at the end of the first lesson. He looked upright, stalwart and erect. I could not believe my eyes.

When he came for his second lesson a couple of days later, he was slumped down again. By the end of this lesson he had again made dramatic changes.

This continued lesson after lesson—enormous postural changes during the lesson, relapses in between lesson. After a couple of weeks, Henry and I became more friendly and conversational. I learned from him that he was a heavy smoker of pot and hashish. He told me he smoked marijuana every night, occasionally in the morning as well, with hashish sometimes substituted for the pot.

Then one day he informed me he had to leave town for a while. He had been convicted of a drug charge and was being sent to a prison farm. Henry called me nine months later when he returned to New York, and he resumed his lessons twice a week. He told me that now he did not smoke frequently, only occasionally. Henry was not as responsive now in each lesson as he used to be. He made appreciably good changes in a lesson, but not as dramatic as before. However, *now he maintained his gains*. There was no relapse between lessons. Instead of one step forward and one backward, he made steady progress. We were both very pleased, and after a few weeks we were satisfied that he could terminate his lessons and maintain his renewed self.

This experience brought a realization to me that substances cannot be substituted for primal thought. Henry was smoking what he thought was a relaxation substance, one that would bring him an escape from the past, future and present.

But it seems that the relaxing the substance was bringing was not a true relaxation. It was a giving up. Pot was an escape. When he lit up, he gave up. He slumped. He let go not only of the past and the future, but the present as well. He collapsed.

A few years later, when I had taught additional students who "smoked" frequently, I received confirmation that Henry's case was not unique. They responded beautifully in the lesson, then regressed quickly in between classes. Marijuana was a powerful mind-body experience, but it was not conducive to learning and maintaining the gains.

➡️ ### The Sights And Sounds
That Speak Books About You

In previous chapters I have made frequent reference to the shape of things past, and how our heavy experiences load and misshape our bodies. Perhaps now it is easier to accept that. Not only is our own body posture affected by these experiences, but subtle characteristics are also present that a skilled Alexander teacher can detect and pin on the past, like skin conditions, the texture of the hair, the sound of the voice. The way a person dresses, the food a person eats, the book a person reads are all a contribution to the sum total of the past.

The more traumatic an experience, the more easily are its effects detected. I have frequently been shown family albums when a student wants to share something of his or her past life with me. I can see in the picture signs of major life events.

"This is right after your mother died."

"Yes, how did you know?"

"I see the tension in your face, and your body started to droop."

"This is while you were starting your new business."

"Let me think. Yes, that's right."

There are other changes, such as in the voice. The voice reflects a great deal and it is now realized that voice tapes audio-analyzed are as unique as fingerprints. They can be used like the polygraph, or lie detector equipment, to detect an increase in tension when a person says something. Just as I take before and after photographs, I may one day make before and after voice tapes. The changes that take place in speaking timbre and inflection are pronounced to my ears, and usually to the ears of the student.

The voice of any tense or habitually uptight person tends not only to be higher-pitched, but it does not project as well. Tension in the neck and throat can produce a higher, tighter voice.

As the body is freed, so are the vocal chords. The voice becomes more resonant, and speech more harmonious. Breathing becomes more rhythmical and this is evident in smoother tones of the voice.

Singers who have taken Alexander lessons for reasons that had no direct connection to their voice, have found to their surprise a vast improvement in their singing voice. I have watched singers and observed their use. At a moment when a singer sings sharp or flat, I can see exactly what he or she is doing with the body at that instant that interferes with his or her good use, and simultaneously interferes with his or her voice. With a singer or actor who has less than ideal voice production, I can see a pattern of poor use in the body. As an Alexander teacher, I also know what can be done to reverse the process from poor use to good use, from a tight voice to a free voice.

There are voice teachers who recognize that posture is interconnected with voice: "Improve your posture and your singing will improve," they say to some of their students. Those who know of the Alexander Technique refer their students for lessons, and soon, there are no more complaints.

I remember one singer who was referred to me for lessons for general improvement. He was a baritone. He was head of the Opera Department of a well-known University. The day he came for his first lesson, he was not feeling well as he had a bad cold. His voice was nasal, light, and tight. He apologized for the way he sounded. I gave him his first lesson, just as I did to any other student who came for his first session. By the end of the lesson, he was aware that his voice had changed. It was deeper, more resonant, and he barely sounded nasal. Before leaving, he walked around the room vocalizing, again and again. He walked around several times, then turned to me and said, "This is remarkable! I came in with this cold, I was nasal, my voice wasn't the way it usually is, it was tight and closed; now, after one lesson, my voice is open and free and my vocalizing is normal, the way it usually is. I tried to vocalize earlier this morning and it was terrible. I'm so enormously impressed that I want to get a government grant to have the Alexander Technique included in the training of opera singers in my department and also at my summer school."

➡ The Whispered Ah-h and Breathing

Alexander did include a breathing technique in his lessons, which he called the "Whispered Ah-h." Breathing techniques are not an essential part of our teaching, as we find that breathing improves automatically as alignment of the body improves. However, Alexander's "Whispered Ah-h" is a very helpful experience.

The student is first asked while directing, to think of smiling, or to actually smile. This brings about a release of tension in the face. The student is then helped by the teacher to bring the lower jaw forward to jut out beyond the upper teeth, and then, while jutting forward like that, and with the aid of Alexander directions, the teacher helps the student open the jaw in a free and easy movement. The student is then asked to gently whisper "ah-h." Then the jaw is allowed to close by itself.

The jaw is "taught" to open and close effortlessly. Lengthening is directed on both the exhalation and inhalation, overcoming the tendency of some to tense up on the inhalation and to collapse down on the exhalation. The diaphragm and ribs begin to work more easily. Together with constant directing, the process is "naturalized." The Whispered Ah-h is usually done with the student sitting on a chair, although some teachers prefer to teach it initially while the student is lying on the table, as that is easier. Whispering "ah" is just the same as saying "ah" for the doctor, except that it is whispered, as if it is a secret.

I would like to show you how you can move your own jaw forward and down and whisper "ah" by yourself, without the help of a teacher. Sit comfortably on a chair, your feet and legs comfortably apart, and your hands resting easily on your thighs. Open your mouth as wide as possible, and close it again. Do this two or three times. Notice how far you open your mouth. Close your mouth.

I would like you to be aware that when you open your mouth you are moving only your lower jaw. Your upper jaw does not move when you open your mouth. Your upper jaw is a fixed part of your skull, whereas your lower jaw is attached to your skull at the jaw joints, which are like hinges, near the lower earlobes. The act of opening your mouth is really the act of moving your *lower jaw downwards*, and closing your mouth is the act of moving your *lower jaw upwards* to meet the upper jaw.

Now jut your lower jaw forward, so that your lower teeth go beyond your upper teeth, and back to normal again. Do this two or three times. Jut it forward and bring it back to neutral. When you jut your lower jaw forward like this, you will feel the jaw muscles that we are usually not aware of. Most of us are holding our jaw muscles with too much work, resulting in too much tension. Very few people have their jaw muscles too slack, where the jaw hangs open all the time.

Move your lower jaw forward about three more times, and then leave your mouth closed. Perhaps what feels normal to you now is different from what felt normal a few minutes ago. Does anything feel freer around your jaw?

Let us develop this movement of moving the jaw forward to bring us to the "Whispered Ah" that is used in the Alexander Technique. Again, jut your lower jaw forward, and while it is forward, open it wide, *gently* keeping the lower jaw *slightly forward*, all the time. When your jaw is open like this, it is forward and down. When you are ready to exhale, whisper "ah-h." As you finish whispering "ah," allow your jaw to close gently, as if it is *floating upwards* to meet your upper jaw. Do this three or four times, freely and gently and easily.

When you open your jaw and again when you whisper "ah," *please* be sure that you are *not* jerking your head backwards, even slightly. All the while, leave your head in a forward and up direction with a slight downward nod. You lower your forehead *slightly* as if you are nodding yes to someone, and you stay in the yes nod. Remember, this is a *slight* nod, not a big movement. It prevents you from throwing your head backwards.

It is essential to add the Alexander directions to the "Whispered Ah-h"! Do the "Whispered Ah-h" three or four more times, and as you do it, tell yourself, "let the neck be free to let the head go forward and up to let the back lengthen and widen." Give your lengthening directions when you move your jaw forwards and downwards, give your lengthening directions again while you whisper "ah," and give them once again while you allow your jaw to float upwards to meet your upper jaw. *Give the directions before, during, and after.*

After having done the "Whispered Ah-h" a few times, see if you feel different. What is your breathing like now? How does your jaw feel? How are you sitting? Is there perhaps some change in the way you sit? Do you feel that you are sitting with greater ease? Move upwards to standing and walk around the room. Do you feel an additional amount of lightness and ease in your walking?

The "Whispered Ah-h" helps improve the breathing. It also gives the experience of exhaling with ease, while lengthening, and inhaling with ease and with lengthening, without effort. While doing the "Whispered Ah-h" the inhalation happens by itself, which is what occurs in good breathing.

In normal daily activities, deep breathing is quiet, soft breathing, and the air comes in by itself through your nostrils. You do not need to "take in" air. This is what you experienced while you were letting your lower jaw gently float upwards to meet your upper jaw. The air was coming in through your nostrils.

When people misuse themselves, they push upwards and tighten when they inhale, and they collapse downwards when they exhale. You might want to feel this. Exaggerate inhaling and exhaling, and I think you will find that as you exaggerate your inhalation, your body pushes up tightly, and as you exaggerate your exhalation, your body collapses as if it wants to fall down. After having done that, it would be a good idea to do a couple of "Whispered Ah-hs" again with good direction to recapture the good experience.

You can do your "Whispered Ah-hs" any time you like. You might be saying to yourself, "Well, when I am at a party, I would look very odd sticking my jaw forward and down and whispering 'ah.' I'll be a laughing stock." Let me tell you how to do it. You can do it *in your imagination*. In your imagination, you smile, move your jaw forwards and downwards while directing "forward and up" and in your imagination you whisper "Ah." After you have become accustomed to that, you can eliminate some of the steps. In your imagination, you could think only of opening your mouth, whispering an "ah," and allowing your mouth to close. It is very helpful when you are in a tense situation, or when you are feeling angry or irritated. It is an effective way to calm yourself. Just do "Whispered Ah-hs" in your imagination.

It is easier to do "Whispered Ah-hs" when lying down.

Lie down on a firm surface with books under your head supporting your head. Gently draw up one knee and then the other knee, so that you are lying with your knees bent, your feet and legs fairly wide apart. When you do your "Whispered Ah-hs" lying down, jutting the lower jaw forward means that it goes up towards the ceiling. And, most important of all, direct "neck free, head forward and out, back lengthening."

I do want to remind you that *all these motions are to be done gently*. When you jut your jaw forward, do not push it to its fullest extent and cause strain. *Jut it forward gently*. Go *almost* to your fullest extent, but not quite. When you open your jaw, do not put effort in trying to keep it forward, do it more through thought, *thinking* of it staying forward as you open your jaw. When you whisper "ah," do not force it out, *allow* it to come out softly and gently as you softly whisper "ah," and then softly allow your jaw to close. You will find that it is easier to do "Whispered Ah-hs" lying down, and I recommend that you first do them this way and then do them while sitting.

When lying down, you can do the Whispered Ah-s with a better chance of maintaining your length. Add your Alexander directions: at each step of your Whispered Ah-h, gently tell your head to go out towards the wall behind you and tell your back and your neck to lengthen following your head. Give those thoughts when you bring your jaw forward, when you bring your jaw forwards and downwards, when you let the air out, when you are whispering your "ah," and again, when you allow the jaw to float closed. And, again, after your jaw is closed and before you bring your jaw forward. Give your directions before, during, and after each movement.

A variation on the Whispered Ah-h, while lying down, could go like this: while lying down with knees bent, open your mouth wide, as if you are going to take a bite out of an apple, whisper ah-h, close your mouth and swallow your saliva. You could repeat this a few times. Notice that the air automatically flows into you, via your nostrils, when you swallow your saliva, and when you open your mouth you are automatically exhaling as you whisper ah-h. You inhale and exhale easily and naturally this way without paying any attention to breathing. After you have done this a few times, lower your legs gently one at a time, close your eyes, and see if the Whispered Ah-h has had an effect on your whole body. Perhaps you are feeling something nicer in your body as you lie here.

When you feel ready to move from here, gently draw up your knees and roll to one side onto your hands and knees and slowly come up to standing. How do you feel as you stand? Walk around the room, and see whether the "Whispered Ah-h" has brought some change into your whole body. Notice your breathing. Is your breathing soft, quiet, and almost not noticeable? Good breathing is soft, quiet, and harmonious, and perhaps you are experiencing that now.

➡ You Learn to Face Life

Just as the body speaks books, so have books been written about body language. It is not my intent to duplicate this coverage, except to say that there is an extensive vocabulary of body language which is perceived and understood by Alexander teachers. We have not been taught to analyze this body language in terms of personality. We do not "read" character; instead, we "read" use; we can see *what a person is doing* that has brought him to his present state and is reinforcing it. And we can show him a way out.

We receive clues about the person from the slightest movements and positions. You, too, receive these clues but the channels of communication are not as open for you as for us. Perhaps you feel uncomfortable with a certain person but you do not know why. So you say that person has bad "vibes." We can see in detail how and where such a person is constricting his body and thus constricting the flow of good "vibes."

You may not always draw an accurate conclusion from a clue. You may be aware of a person not looking at you while talking, for instance, and conclude that such a person is shifty, or not to be trusted, when in actuality that person may be totally trustworthy but not ready to confront people, or even life, itself.

As one Alexander student put it, "In an approach where you learn to be forward and up and to look straight ahead, you learn to face life."

So it is that through the Alexander lessons, the way a person reacts in everyday social intercourse becomes more pleasant and direct. Subliminally, others pick this up. As you improve through Alexander you come across to other people in more positive and acceptable ways. And they respond differently to you.

This is an area where details and particulars are difficult to pinpoint through example. But time and time again, failure-prone people become successful, and unpopular people become well-liked.

"You've changed. But I can't say what it is."

"You have been doing something different. You seem so improved."

"You appear so much happier than when I last saw you."

This is the kind of feedback students report receiving from their friends and acquaintances.

From doing the few movements provided in this book and repeating the directions over and over to yourself during the day, you could begin to get similar feedback.

"You look taller." "You seem more energetic." "You have more poise." "You move more smoothly."

As you become better balanced, you become less rigid. Emotions play across your face. You become more vital, more expressive, more alive. The "masks" drop off, the armoring melts away, and the real you radiates to others.

Whatever your excess, it normalizes. The excessively rigid becomes softer, the hyperactive becomes calmer, the sluggish becomes more vital. You are brought to a more natural state, the natural state of man is a state of joy.

Chapter 9

Comparisons, Contrasts, and Similarities of Other Approaches

Reichian Therapy and the Alexander Technique

WHEN PEOPLE LEARN that I have been involved in Reichian therapy, they are interested to know if it is similar to Alexander work.

Although there is some similarity in philosophy, the two are totally dissimilar in approach. Reichian therapy stemmed from psychoanalysis, Wilhelm Reich having been a disciple of Freud's. He realized, as he worked with his patients, that more progress was effected when he encouraged them to breathe deeply, which led to their becoming more in touch with their feelings; and to use the body to manifest emotions, rather than just talk about them, as with rage, fear, grief and joy. As the emotions were released and expressed, there was a corresponding softening of the muscular rigidity.

Deep breathing is the basic part of Reichian therapy, and it leads, sooner or later, to emotional release during the therapy sessions. During the sessions, the patient lies on a couch, partially undressed, and with knees bent. The release of emotions can involve kicking and hitting the couch, screaming, shouting, sobbing, and laughter. Sensations are often experienced internally by the patient as "streamings." The therapy is designed to lead people to becoming more open, free-flowing and better-functioning in love, work, and knowledge.

In the Alexander lessons, we work differently. Our work is not a therapy, it is an education, or, more accurately, a reeducation. I cannot deny that many of the benefits are therapeutic, but we do not approach our work as a matter of treating a problem; we approach it as a matter of teaching improved use. We work with the use of the body, and as the body tensions soften, the person becomes more open and expressive.

Muscular blocks are released in Reichian therapy through deep breathing and expressing emotions, and in Alexander lessons through ease of motion under mental directions. By dissolving the muscular blocks, or "armoring," via either method, changes are effected in the personality. The two methods can bring about some of the same results, and also each method brings something different. I do not believe that Alexander is as effective as Reichian therapy in working with emotions, nor is Reichian therapy as effective as Alexander in bringing about a freer body. The combination of the two methods is superb; where a person's resistance in one method is too powerful to be dissolved, the other method may dissolve it. More layers of the onion are peeled away than with one method alone; more layers of rigidity, armoring, defensiveness, self-protection and muscular tension are dissolved. Both Reich and Alexander believed that were more people improved by their own method, the world would become a place of open, loving people and there would be no more war.

I have seen people go through both Reichian therapy and Alexander lessons with excellent results. The procedures do not clash or interfere, they supplement each other, one focusing on body, the other on emotion.

➡ How Does Bio-Energetics Compare?

Bio-energetics, another "body psychotherapy" that has become widely used today, is an offshoot of Reichian therapy. It was founded by Alexander Lowen, a former Reichian therapist. He developed his own version of the work.

Bio-energetics differs from Reichian work in its thrust toward physical exercises that encourage deep breathing and the ensuing emotional release. Lowen added group work in addition to individual work. In my opinion, the comparison between Bio-energetics and the Alexander Technique is the same as the comparison with Reichian therapy.

➡️ Gestalt Therapy and the Alexander Technique

Gestalt therapy was founded by Fritz Perls. It is more verbally oriented than Reichian therapy and Bio-energetics.

In Gestalt, both spoken language and body language play a large role. Perls developed a different verbal approach than the classical method used in psychoanalysis, as well as a different approach to dream analysis. His method also takes into account what the body is "saying" when spoken words are expressed.

For instance, if the patient is sitting on a chair talking about his job and is drumming on the arm of the chair with his fingers, the therapist may begin to work in some way with that movement. This apparently insignificant act could lead to some more significant physical movement and/or to an important insight on the part of both the therapist and patient. Gestalt therapy also encourages free expression of emotions.

Ego, Hunger and Aggression, written by Fritz Perls some thirty-five years ago when he was living and practicing in South Africa, was his first book on Gestalt therapy. It outlines his ideas and how he arrived at them. He makes frequent reference to Alexander and his work, and quotes from Alexander's books.

Gestalt, like Alexander, is concerned with being in the present, in the "here and now," as compared to methods of psychotherapy that are more concerned with the "why," a "past"-related approach, and therapies that are future-oriented.

Gestalt and Alexander work are both concerned with how the person presents himself, how he behaves, how he communicates, and how he uses his body. A great degree of the past surfaces in this process, but the thrust is in the "here and now" and Fritz Perls is largely credited with that concept.

In *Ego, Hunger and Aggression*, Fritz Perls acknowledges Alexander's concepts of "means whereby" and "end-gaining" as the source of his work dealing with staying in the "here and now" as compared to being "goal-oriented." This illustrates the link between the two approaches. While we who teach the Alexander lessons do not work psychologically with people, we do work with a mind-body unity. The mind and the body are used, the two working together, leading to greater awareness and improvement. In Gestalt, the mind is used in broader ways; the physical is used in working with what a movement is expressing. The Gestalt therapist does not put his hands on the patient to teach better ways of movement. He does, however, lead a patient to new ways of thinking and being, and awareness.

I have known Alexander students who progress faster than other people in the Gestalt work, and the same is true for many Gestalt patients who have taken Alexander lessons.

▶ Feldenkrais and Alexander

Alexander and Feldenkrais are often mentioned in the same breath, and often written about at the same time as the two prime examples of a psychophysical approach to reeducation. These two methods are singled out as teaching a reeducation, as compared to giving a treatment; and involving mind and body in both method and results; they bring deep changes in the body which also affect personality. These two methods are closest in approach to each other than any of the other methods, and yet there are differences. The philosophy behind the approach is almost identical in both methods.

Dr. Moshe Feldenkrais, the Russian-Israeli former physicist and Judo champion who forty-five years ago founded the method that is named after him, has developed two different approaches. One is called *Awareness Through Movement*, and the other is *Functional Integration*.

Functional Integration was first developed by Moshe Feldenkrais while he was in the process of finding a way to cure his severely injured knee that threatened to prevent him from walking for the rest of his life. Functional Integration is individual work, where the Feldenkrais practitioner works on the body of a student, while the student is passive. The work is more manipulative than in Alexander, works with various parts of the body, and is done in silence. The student lies, clothed, in a variety of positions—lying down on the back, on the front, or on the side, or kneeling, sitting or standing. Although the Feldenkrais teacher does not use the words used in the Alexander Technique, he or she has been trained to work with length and with good direction in his or her own body. Functional Integration brings about great improvement in alignment and functioning, and is also very successful in working with physical ailments, both minor and major, including multiple sclerosis and celebral palsy. Dr. Feldenkrais has stated that in general a person should have one Functional Integration lesson per year of his life, so that generally a twenty-year-old would require twenty lessons and a forty-year-old would require forty lessons. Although it can be of benefit to everyone, the remarkable results achieved with severe ailments makes it highly recommendable in such cases.

Functional Integration and the Alexander Technique both work on an individual basis, although the actual methods are different from each other. Some people have reported more progress with one, and others have reported more progress with the other. An excellent program would be to have lessons in both Functional Integration and the Alexander Technique.

Dr. Feldenkrais continued to develop his work so that it could reach a larger number of people, and he invented movements and exercises that would duplicate what is done in the Functional Integration lessons. He has called this approach Awareness Through Movement. Over the years, he has developed over three thousand lessons, and each lesson includes several different types of movements. Much of his work is inspired by the Alexander Technique, Yoga, Judo, Sufi dances, the Gindler Method, and other disciplines. The variety and depth of understanding behind Dr. Feldenkrais' work is ingenious. Dr. Feldenkrais' understanding of the cause-effect relationship of brain and body is unique, and has brought him to evolve a unique system of exercises. Most of the exercises are done lying on the floor, usually on the back; however, there are many variations, such as lying on the stomach, lying on the side, sitting in different positions, kneeling, crawling, and standing. The Awareness Through Movement instructor does not work individually with people in the class, nor demonstrate. The students are to discover the movements for themselves, so that the learning comes from within and therefore is better integrated. The types of movements vary greatly in range from tiny movements to large acrobatic movements: sometimes there is no movement, and only the imagination is used to bring changes into the body. There are movements that are unique, originating with Dr. Feldenkrais; there are others that are recognizable from yoga, judo or calisthenics, but the manner of teaching them is uniquely Feldenkrais: they are taught without strain, effortlessly, without trying to reach a goal, and often through doing different movements that seem to have no connection with the original movement. The Feldenkrais approach is slow, gentle, and occasionally fast; playful or meditative; using constant awareness of *how* one is moving and *where* the change is taking place; doing less rather than doing more—doing few movements, and doing smaller movements than one is capable of. "Do less than what you can do" is a common Feldenkrais instruction.

Dancers, yoga teachers, physical education teachers and their students, are all astonished at the additional limberness they achieve through these gentle, nonrepetitive unusual movements. Feldenkrais' Awareness Through Movement brings to many people a suppleness that they never dreamed was possible for them. In addition, there are changes that correspond to some of the changes from the Alexander Technique; a reeducation in alignment and functioning. Dr. Feldenkrais talks of teaching the nervous system through the means of the body, and the nervous system is involved with all areas of our life.

Awareness Through Movement is not suitable for those who are in such severe pain that they cannot lie down on the floor. However, it has been successful in alleviating many lesser pains, aches and disabilities.

I have seen Awareness Through Movement and the Alexander Technique bring about some of the same results, and I also see that each one can give more to a person in a particular direction. The Alexander Technique can bring a person further along the path of a daily, lasting change on a very deep level; and Awareness Through Movement can take a person further along the path of a suppleness beyond the ordinary.

The combination of Alexander and Feldenkrais is very exciting and rewarding, and is highly recommended by many people.

➡ Rolfing and the Alexander Technique

People often ask about the difference between Rolfing and the Alexander Technique. Both methods have a powerful effect on posture.

Rolfing was developed by Ida Rolf, who lived into her eighties. It is a method of intense body manipulative massage which is often called a deep tissue massage. In most cases, it is quite painful. Another term for Rolfing is Structural Integration.

In Rolfing, the client lies on the floor, wearing underwear or a swimsuit. The Rolfer applies the hands, knuckles and elbows with considerable pressure to different parts of the body. Each of the first ten sessions is devoted to a different part of the body. The whole body is covered in the initial ten sessions, or ten hours, but most people take many more than ten sessions.

It is a very effective method to obtain improved alignment. Rolfing works on the connective tissue connecting muscle to muscle and muscle to bone. According to Ida Rolf, this connective tissue has shortened when a body has poor alignment.

The Rolfer, through deep penetration, is releasing and stretching the connective tissue, with a resulting release in the musculature.

Many people who have been Rolfed have experienced emotional releases during their sessions and claim that it has improved their emotional lives. They have experienced deep feelings from the past surfacing during a Rolfing treatment as the traumas of yesterday, still etched into the cells, are released. This does not happen with everyone who is Rolfed.

The similarity between Rolfing and the Alexander Technique is certainly not apparent in the hands—one is painful pressure, the other a feathery touch. But, basically, the aim of improved body functioning is the same, leading to higher levels of health and well-being.

The major difference is that Rolfing is a treatment, Alexander is a reeducation.

With Rolfing, the posture is changed through severe pressure, and as a result, the way a person moves is usually improved. My conversations with people who have been Rolfed, as well as with Rolfers, give me the impression that there are certain types of people who do not respond well to this method; those who do, experience excellent results.

Rolfers work on one part of the body and then another, until eventually the whole body is corrected; they change the whole through working on the parts. Alexander teachers work on the whole body, teaching how to move in an improved way, the individual parts change as the whole body improves and comes into a better alignment.

In Rolfing, the alignment is changed as a means to good motion. In Alexander, good motion is taught as a means to improve alignment.

Participation is another difference. In Rolfing, the Rolfer does the work, and works hard, while the client lies still. In Alexander, the student and teacher work together, as effortlessly as possible, in the activities of daily life, and mental directions are used by the student both during lessons and at other times for self-help.

There is a great deal of similarity between Rolfing and Alexander in the improvement of the postural alignment. A partnership between the two has been found to be excellent: those who have been Rolfed are usually more ready for Alexander and responsive to it than many others; and many of those who have been Alexandered are found by Rolfers to be easier to work with and there is less pain. Each method can do something that the other cannot do. One method reinforces the other, and progress goes further when a person has experienced both Rolfing and Alexander.

▶ Is Chiropractics Similar to Alexander?

The similarity between Chiropractics and the Alexander Technique is that both methods have the understanding that the well-being of the body is dependent on the condition of the spine. Both methods understand that the good alignment of the back, and the spine, is essential for the body to function well, to prevent backaches, slipped discs, muscle spasm and many other ailments that may or may not seem to be directly connected to the spine and back. The approach is very different.

Chiropractics is a treatment. For many injuries it can be essential to go to a chiropractor; for example, if a bone is out of place, or vertebrae are dislocated, a good chiropractor can take care of such problems well. Their work, which is strongly manipulative of the spine, is always in the direction of improved alignment.

However, in ailments where muscular misuse is the major culprit, the chiropractic work of realigning the spine often brings only temporary relief. There are many conditions of aches and pains, particularly back problems and neck problems, that are not actually alleviated by chiropractics, but do get temporary relief after each session, and prevent worsening of the condition. The person often becomes dependent on going to the chiropractor.

The Alexander Technique is not a treatment, it is a reeducation that teaches people how to function in the best possible way with the least amount of muscular tension. Because of the improved use, the better functioning and the release of tension on the problem areas, pain is usually relieved, on a lasting basis, and the student becomes independent of the Alexander teacher.

Alexander teachers have had many cases of people who came for Alexander lessons who were going regularly to a chiropractor and after a short while found that they no longer needed the chiropractor. On the other hand, I have occasionally referred an Alexander student to a good chiropractor for assistance in an area that was not relieved through Alexander.

▶ The Martial Arts and the Alexander Technique

The Oriental martial arts are enjoying a surge of Western interest that parallels the recognition of mind-body unity. These include Karate, Judo, Aikido, and T'ai chi.

In most of these, particularly T'ai chi and Aikido, there is great emphasis on energy flow and how it is directed by the mind. This is expressed by T'ai chi Master Cheng Man-ch'ing when he writes,* "What is meant by the correct method of body and function? The answer is that the mind commands and the body obeys. Remember well the chief purpose: the rejuvenation and prolongation of life."

"Holding the head as if suspended by a string from above, the

---

*T'ai Chi, by Cheng Man-ch'ing and Robert W. Smith, Charles E. Tuttle Co., Rutland, Vermont, 1967.

entire body feels light and nimble." Alexander? No, Master Cheng.

"The mind leads and the body follows." Again, it could be Alexander speaking, but it is the T'ai chi master.

The mind directs the *chi*, life energy, and properly directed, it circulates throughout the body, and vitality levels rise. An erect and relaxed body is conducive to this circulation, says Master Cheng, and that is when body clumsiness and heaviness is replaced with the grace and ease that makes the head appear to be suspended by a string from above.

People who take lessons in T'ai chi find that changes also take place in their emotional well-being. The lovely flow that is experienced while proceeding through T'ai chi positions is quite similar to that experienced with the directions of the Alexander Technique. Both are gentle and effortless. Both require good use of the head, neck and back to allow legs and arms to move smoothly and lightly.

T'ai chi is said to have started out as a boxing technique for self-defense, but it evolved into a discipline of the mind and body with a wide spectrum of benefits from its 108 movements.

These movements flow one into the other and are performed gently and slowly. Patterned after animal movements and other movements found in nature, they attune the mind to life energy, thus benefiting both mind and body.

Some forms of T'ai chi use faster movements, but they are always flowing. A superiority of body use and mental agility is claimed as well as improved health that can add twenty years to one's life.

The third dimension of man—his spirit—is affected, along with the body and mind. A feeling of oneness with nature, with the very cosmos, is frequently reported; it is this feeling that we interpret as the most striking clue that what is at work in T'ai chi is also at work in the Alexander Technique.

A major difference between T'ai chi and Alexander is that, to get the full benefits in T'ai chi, it is necessary to maintain a strict schedule of practice, twice a day, morning and evening, for the rest of one's days. Without practicing, even though it has been thoroughly and proficiently learned, one does not profit from the benefits. In the Alexander Technique, there is no practice time necessary in addition to the lessons, and eventually not even the lessons are necessary.

While the "delicious" feeling might be similar, it is not as permanent as in Alexander, unless one has practiced for some years, although it is recapturable. With many people, the "flow" of T'ai chi does not flow over into their daily lives, it is experienced only during and immediately after the T'ai chi lesson or practice.

I have been a student of T'ai chi and I love it. I get a feeling of joy from it. However, not only was this feeling of joy less lasting than in Alexander, it was also less universal. Most of my fellow students in class learned to improve their use while doing the T'ai chi movements, and when the class was over, they reverted to their former tense posture and tight movements and continued their daily life this way.

The daily practice of T'ai chi, however, would recapture temporarily the beneficial flow and ease for these people and that in itself brought improvements in their bodies and alleviated some of their ailments.

I have had three or four Aikido lessons. This martial art focuses more on the art of defense then, as karate might, on attack. The skills emphasize throwing the opponent off balance and thus defending yourself successfully against an attack. Here, more than in Judo and Karate, the mind is used to direct the body. In this regard, it comes a step closer to Alexander.

The Master in the Aikido class I attended would test students periodically during the lesson to see if they were using their mind to direct their body. In one of the tests, while the student is standing arms at side, the Master grasps the right wrist, holds it down, and asks the student to raise that arm. When the student tries to lift the arm with physical effort, it does not move. When the student does as taught and uses his mind, saying to himself, "I am going to raise my right arm," he finds he can raise it.

In another test the Master lines the class up next to a wall, standing sideways with their right palm against the wall. He then goes from one to the other trying to pull the hand away from the wall. If he can do it, it indicates that the student was using physical effort to keep the hand there. If he cannot, the student was giving himself mental directions like, "My hand is going through the wall to the other side." These mental directions are powerful.

In another test, the Master would ask the class to stand with their knees bent. He would go from student to student and try to push each one over. If they lost balance, the mind was not being used properly. Those who directed their balance with their mind were not "pushovers."

Both Aikido and Alexander use the mind to direct the body. Another similarity is the stance they use, and the alignment of the back. The back has to be solid, well-integrated, and in a natural, erect posture. This is common to *all* of the martial arts. Also, their stance has the knees bent, reminiscent of our own teaching of bending the knees rather than the back as proper use in bending, and this allows the intrinsic power of the back muscles to be functioning fully—it gives good balance and strength to the whole body.

Judo and Karate also require a solid, well-integrated back to give power to the movements of arms and legs, and to provide a solid balance. Through this balance, they acquire the agility to move extremely fast, with skill and power.

Those who are expert in these martial arts are a superb example of good use of the body, and without that excellent use, one could not achieve the greatest skill in these arts.

Unfortunately, many students of the martial arts learn how to move well, with good, free use of their bodies, only while practicing their particular art, and are not taught to have this good use in their daily lives. As far as I can tell, these people would never become great masters of the art.

The masters I have seen in T'ai chi, Aikido, Judo and Karate, whether in the flesh or on film, all moved superbly in every activity of their body. Often, they do not know how to impart this quality on a constant level to their students. This is where Alexander can be an excellent adjunct to the martial arts, and teach people how to achieve greater heights of body skill in their life as well as in the skills of martial arts.

▶ Bio-Feedback as a Teaching Device

Electronic devices that measure pulse, temperature, blood pressure, muscular movement, brain wave cycles, and skin resistance are now connected to visual and audio circuits which, through their flashing lights and beeping noises, provide signals to the user of changes in their functioning.

Bio-feedback is a useful teaching device. If you think of a peaceful scene and a light flashes indicating that your blood pressure has dropped, then you have learned a way to normalize high blood pressure through mental direction.

At the Menninger Clinic in Topeka, Kansas, it was found that if a person could learn to make his hands hot, his headache would disappear. How do you go about mentally raising the temperature of your hands? It is not to be found in the how-to books. So, you hold the bio-feedback thermal units and do mentally what you think might raise the temperature of your hands.

One person might get an immediate response by thinking about his hands as surrounded by a red color. Another person may get a good response imagining his hands in a tub of intensely hot water.

Direct control over the autonomic nervous system can be acquired through this bio-feedback way of learning. A person can learn to control not only headaches and blood pressure, but pulse and movement of the bowels as well.

Bio-feedback has become accepted to the extent that prominent medical institutions are researching it and medical schools are teaching it.

Areas of research include:

- Ulcers and digestive tract ailments, in which the patient learns to slow stomach and intestinal contractions.
- Impotency, a fairly new area, but one in which men are successfully learning to regain erections.
- Alcohol, drug dependency, and addiction; while not cured, the withdrawal symptoms are controlled.
- Phobias, handled by conditioning not to respond to certain stimuli with fears and stress.
- Muscle rehabilitation (retraining the muscles), for patients who have suffered partial paralysis through stroke or accident.

What has bio-feedback got to do with the Alexander Technique? As as Alexander teacher, I am a bio-feedback device. I provide human bio-feedback rather than auditory or visual feedback. Between me and the full-length mirror, another visual feedback device, the student has the advantages of a bio-feedback laboratory.

The electromyograph (EMG) measures the slightest tendency to move a muscle even before the actual motion has gotten under way. The hands of the Alexander teacher pick up these impulses just as sensitively as the electromyograph. After three years of training, it becomes second nature.

The brain encephalograph (EEG) measures the rapidity of brain pulsations. You and I have these pulsations at a rate of 14 to 21 per second while in the normal awake state, called beta. As we relax, these pulsations slow down to 7 to 14 pulsations per second to a state called alpha. If you were giving yourself mental directions in an Alexander lesson and you suddenly became tense because you were physically exerting yourself, the EEG would register an increase in brain waves, possibly informing you that you moved from alpha to beta.

However, you do not need the EEG or the EMG in an Alexander lesson because the Alexander teacher would also signal you that your brain waves were increasing or your muscles tightening by saying, "You're contracting."

When we say mind-body unity, we are not saying only that the mind controls the body, but also that the body controls the mind. The two are indivisible. The two are cause and effect. They work as an inseparable unit. Change one and you alter the other. Some of the ailments that have reportedly responded to bio-feedback, such as headaches, digestive tract ailments and muscle rehabilitation, have also responded to the Alexander Technique.

I would venture to say that with the Alexander Technique one has learned to reeducate more of one's body in many more areas than would happen with a bio-feedback device. However, bio-feedback has been effective in cases of specific ailments that may not have been affected by Alexander lessons.

We see here equally successful mind-body approaches emphasizing the body or the mind, and I have seen people in pain develop greater control over their involuntary system by combining bio-feedback with the Alexander Technique.

➡ Bates Vision Improvement and Alexander

The Bates method* of vision improvement, and its later refinement known as the Bates-Corbett method, is based on a re-education of how you use your eyes and the muscles around them. I took lessons in both the Bates method and Bates-Corbett, and both teachers called my progress "incredibly fast," which I attribute to the mind-body communications already established through Alexander lessons.

My teacher of the Bates-Corbett Method, Janet Goodrich, asked for a good deal of fantasizing of images in her training. I found I could do it instantly and easily. Janet was surprised. "You are near-sighted," she said, "and near-sighted people do not fantasize easily." This reminded me that when I was in my teens and early twenties I had had great difficulty when asked to imagine something. "It must be the Alexander Technique," we both said, "that's changed that."

I have found that the Alexander Technique did what I wanted for my body, and the Bates Vision Improvement did what I wanted for my eyes.

Although eye exercises are part of the method, its key is the teaching of relaxed use of the eyes through reeducation of daily habits of seeing. Bates teachers who are most successful use a great deal of mental thoughts to redirect the habitual way people use their eyes to see.

I would say that with such teachers, the Vision Improvement work is the Alexander Technique of eye use.

Among my students I have found that only an occasional one reports better vision through the Alexander Technique. Among Bates vision students, there is an immediate speeding up of vision improvement when they add Alexander lessons to the process. It seems evident that the eyes need their own reeducation, but that it is not always possible to free the eyes without freeing the body.

➡ A Psychosynthesis Workshop

Moving further into the mental end of this spectrum of ap-

---

*Better Eyesight Without Glasses, W.H. Bates, M.D.; Holt, Rhinehart, and Winston, New York, 1940.

proaches, some years ago I participated in a weekend workshop in Psychosynthesis with Robert and Donna Gerard. Here the emphasis was directing one's energy while sitting with eyes closed. There was also much emphasis on fantasizing.

After each directed fantasy, the Gerards asked for feedback from the forty or so participants. We found that I gave this feedback more readily and specifically than the others who had not set up the kind of mental-physical communications that I had through my years of this kind of work. In addition, I not only saw the fantasy I had created, I sensed in my body the feelings connected with it and felt that I was part of it, instead of only being an observer. After describing this, in relation to one of my fantasies, Robert Gerard said: "You have had a cosmic experience."

Whatever you call such an experience, I would not be able to have it were I not "opened" to it by my body-mind training.

Those of you who have done the simple exercises in this book and who continue to use mental directions to maintain good use of the body, are paving the way for this mind-body avenue of communication to ecstatic joy in the workshop called Life.

➡ The Mind Courses, Hypnotism,
and The Alexander Technique

EST (Erhardt Seminars Training) and Silva Mind Control are the two best known of the mind courses, and they both share a lot in common with Science of Mind, hypnotism and other related methods.

Since my writing associate, Robert B. Stone, is an accredited Silva Mind Control lecturer, I have asked him to describe it in his words:

"Briefly, it is a means of getting control of the subconscious and of the superconscious. The subconscious control enables you to consciously control habits, fears, personality quirks and physical problems. The superconscious control enables you to consciously trigger intuition, creativity, and problem-solving ability, often with so-called extrasensory perception and psychic ability very much in evidence.

"It is accomplished through a series of alpha level conditioning cycles that, in effect, actuate the right hemisphere of the brain which operates in the internal environment. This is the non-material realm, the cause of all material effect. So you move from being a victim of circumstances to a creator of circumstances."

The mental pictures you see become quite real in life. Just as you picture the neck free, it becomes free, and as you picture the head forward and up to let the back lengthen and widen, all of these bodily changes do indeed take place. In the mind courses, one is taught to be at the alpha level when creating mental pictures.

Hypnotism and self-hypnotism are also taught in commercial courses. Both are mental approaches to mind-body mastery. Hypnotism uses an operator and a subject; self-hypnotism makes the individual both operator and subject. Here it is the subconscious that is reached for physical and emotional improvement.

When I taught Alexander in New York, one of my students, Juan L., would respond best when he returned from a vacation. He was both a student and a job holder and led a very stressful life in the city. I could always tell when he had taken a few days off because then his body responded very easily to mental instructions.

On one of Juan's best days, I remarked "You have just returned from a vacation."

"Wrong," he responded. "I have had a hypnosis session."

He told me how he had written down the Alexander verbal directions, let the neck be free, to let the head go forward and up, to let the back lengthen and widen, for his hypnotist so that he could be given those directions by her while in the hypnotic state. He certainly had responded excellently to this hypnosis and Alexander coupling.

He went a second time to the hypnotist for further reinforcement, but I could not detect any further improvement in his response, nor could he. We concluded that the hypnotic suggestion had reproduced the best Alexander experience of his lessons, but that it had not taken him beyond that.

He then had the hypnotist teach him self-hypnosis, so he could give himself the Alexander directions as self-hypnotic suggestions. Here, too, we found that the self-hypnosis did no more than help him reexperience his optimum results.

Hypnosis and self-hypnosis can be a useful tool to reinforce Alexander results; however, based on this person's experience, it could neither replace nor extend these results.

Some people who hear that we give mental instructions in the Alexander lessons remark that it is similar to hypnosis or self-hypnosis. Alexander himself was confronted with this, but felt very strongly that his teaching was not related to hypnosis. He pointed out that the lessons are conducted in a wide-awake state, the same state in which the student arrives for his lesson. It is not given in a sleep or semi-trance state as in hypnosis or self-hypnosis. Today's use of the word hypnosis is more broadly interpreted. A television commercial that directs you to buy "Mother's Bread" is today considered a form of hypnotic suggestion.

The similarity between self-hypnosis and the Alexander Technique is that the mind is directing and the body follows the directions. The similarity, as far as I can tell, ends there.

Alexander learning, in my opinion, is more closely aligned to the process of a conditioned response. It is analogous to the way Pavlov's dogs salivated at the sound of the bell, after the bell had been rung a number of instances prior to the dogs' feeding. The words are being mentally said while the teacher's hands are guiding the experience. The words are like the bell. The student can continue giving himself the words and evoke the same improved movement.

Pavlov's dogs were given a respite from the conditioning of the bell, and then it was rung again before each feeding. The second time around the dogs began to salivate at the sound with far fewer repetitions needed than the first time.

Similarly, Alexander students who develop a conditioned response can be restimulated quite easily to that response. Another lesson takes up where the previous one left off. Even after a lapse of time, renewal of the mental direction brings a rapid renewal of the response. Poor habits, too, can be easily restimulated, so the Alexander student needs to use the mental direction to reinforce the restimulation of the good habits. Keeping the eyes open becomes of functional importance in the Alexander lessons. It is not a meditation. It is not a state of mental "not doing"; it is a mental "doing."

In my practice, I experience that when an Alexander student closes the eyes, the direction stops. The "flow" goes dead. In an advanced Alexander student, the closing of the eyes might not cut off the "flow," but it lessens it noticeably.

As an open-eyed conditioned response, the Alexander Technique is a far cry from hypnotism. As Alexander himself said about the values of his teaching, they are " . . .not to be won in sleep, in trance, in submission, in paralysis, or in anesthesia, but in a clear open-eyed reasoning, deliberate consciousness and apprehension of the wonderful potentialities possessed by mankind . . ."

▶ The Benefits of Meditation

Meditation has been around a long time. However, Western civilization has been the last to adopt it. Common to many meditation systems is the repetition of a word, sound or mantra, silently or aloud, usually with the eyes closed and the body in a comfortable sitting position, or in a lotus or a kneeling position.

Meditation, observed under laboratory conditions, has been shown to decrease metabolism, lower blood pressure, slow down the phase brain waves, slow down respiration and pulse, and decrease the body's consumption of oxygen.

Benefits are physical, mental, and spiritual. Two brief periods a day, about 15 minutes each, appear to relieve stress and fatigue, increase energy and efficiency, and produce alertness, tranquility, well-being and inner peace, and a sense of "meditative" flow in the body.

However, I have not heard of TM or other forms of meditation creating a straight back out of a sway back, or correcting the other bodily signs of stress and anxiety. Meditate, if you can, with a wry neck or a pinched nerve.

Bad body use needs to be halted. Good body use needs to be relearned in its place. This is not the domain of meditation, wide as its domain most certainly is. It is the domain of the Alexander Technique.

Many meditators complain that their back or neck hurts so much while meditating that they know they would benefit more from their meditation if they felt more freedom and ease in their bodies. Here again, the Alexander Technique has led people further along the path they have chosen by releasing the obstacles on the way.

The benefits of meditation rely on daily practice. The benefits of the Alexander Technique do not. Through the Alexander Technique one can have some of the benefits of meditation. Combining meditation and the Alexander Technique could be the ultimate answer for many people. Aldous Huxley devoted a whole novel—*Eyeless in Gaza*—to this.

Some Alexander students find they do not require meditation when they have learned the Alexander Technique, as they have learned to have "energy in stillness, and meditation in movement."

▶ Nutrition and The Alexander Technique

Many people have asked: "Does the Alexander Technique include a diet?" The answer is no, it does not. However, many Alexander teachers are personally interested in good nutrition and choose to live on a diet of healthy foods. This is a purely personal choice and is not included in the teaching of the Alexander Technique.

An improved diet can bring many benefits, but it cannot change the habitual use of your body; it does not get rid of slumped shoulders, sway backs, knock knees, and flat feet.

An interesting fact is that the weight of a person is not the factor involved in whether a person feels light or heavy to an Alexander teacher. A 250-lb. person can have excellent upward direction in his or her body and move lightly through the movements, while a scanty 98-lb. person can be rigid and heavy in his or her motions.

I knew a slender young woman who weighed 108 lbs., and I always knew when she was in the house, as her footsteps were heavy and loud; I would hear her stomping through the house as if she were a hefty man wearing hobnailed boots. Needless to say, she had a very swayed back, a stiff neck, and rigid legs. After a few Alexander lessons, she walked so lightly that I could not tell whether she was in the house or not.

I have worked with very slender young children who felt as heavy as a sack of lead, and I have worked with two or three people who weighed 200 lbs. or more who felt light and moved easily.

I have noticed, however, that when a person has been overeating he or she feels heavier and has difficulty moving, regardless of whether he or she is thin or fat. And when a person eats lightly, he or she feels lighter and is more responsive to directions and the teacher's touch.

It is clear that eating heavily makes us heavier and more sluggish, and eating lightly makes us lighter and more buoyant. I have felt and seen similar differences when people have changed from an "unhealthy" diet to a more nourishing one.

A better diet can also improve the tone of the skin and muscles, bring more glow to hair, skin, and eyes, and bring about greater buoyancy and feelings of well-being. But, diet *cannot* alter the movement habits of a lifetime.

Combine a healthy diet with the Alexander Technique and you will be adding a plus to the benefits of the lessons.

➡ Holistic Health

A new school of thought is now emerging. Its umbrella term is "holistic health," sometimes spelled "wholistic." It is the realization of body, mind, and spirit all playing a role in health.

Carl Simonton, M.D., teaches his cancer patients to relax and visualize the body's defense system getting rid of the cancer cells.

Esalan Institute at Big Sur conducts an ongoing program of multifaceted approaches to the perfectability of man.

Holistic health centers and clinics, many organized by physicians, are springing up all oved the country, combining such diverse bedfellows as astrology, palmistry, acupuncture, touch for health, massage, prayer therapy, and nutrition, as well as the methods discussed in this chapter.

These growth centers admit the whole person into their curriculum, incorporating mind, body, emotion and spirit. The mind-body relationship is finally being recognized and incorporated into health, education and psychotherapy.

➡ Relaxation

I would like to talk a little about the word "relaxation." Most people, when asked to relax, do exactly what I had asked you to do when I asked you to slump down. Most people associate the word or the idea of relaxation with hanging downwards, which results in being heavy. What the Alexander Technique gives people is a relaxation of a different kind. Because it is so different to what people usually think of as relaxation, we rarely use the word "relax." However, a term that could describe the results of the Alexander Technique is "dynamic relaxation." With dynamic relaxation your body is light, buoyant, and directed upwards, instead of directed downwards and heavy. And yet, with the Alexander directions, there is a strong feeling of relaxation. This is a relaxation that comes from having let go of tension. As all tension involves excessive shortening and contracting of muscles, when we stop contracting them and they are more lengthened, we feel the relaxation that comes with the release of tension. We feel we are relaxed while being light and going upwards.

Many of these new approaches to mind-body balance make you feel good. However, the good feeling, even a joyous feeling, is not likely to be as fully permeating as the Alexander joy. It is in my experience a more temporary euphoria, analogous to what the athlete experiences after a stimulating game or contest. The cardiovascular system is stimulated and oxygen surges into all the cells of the body. But then a few hours later, or a day or two later, all is back to normal, or abnormal. Nothing has been learned. One has to rely on regular practice, and when one gives that up, too often trouble starts in the mind-body organism as there has been no *real* change.

The Alexander Technique could be taken on its own and bring about great improvements. On the other hand, it can be taken as a jumping-off point; the Technique can open us and free us in a unique way. This opening-up allows us to be far more receptive to any other method that we explore, or any other experience that we have; it could be taken as a foundation for other experiences, for therapy, for learning, for all activities. It opens us up to getting more benefit from anything else we go into. For myself, the Alexander Technique has changed every area of my life. I have found this to be the most valuable thing I have ever done. It has helped me get far more out of everything else that I have done.

I can agree with what many Alexander students say: "I have tried many things, but none of them have done for me what Alexander has done. The Alexander Technique has brought about *the changes that I wanted!*"

Chapter 10

Unveiling the Real You For a Joyous New Life

"EVERY MAN, WOMAN AND CHILD," said Alexander, "holds the possibility of physical perfection; it rests with each of us to attain it by personal understanding and effort."

This is more true than ever before. Rising hospital costs, crowded mental institutions, and inefficient delivery of health care to the public places a larger responsibility on our own shoulders to stay well, physically and mentally.

Thanks to the many alternatives to allopathic medicine that are now riding the wave of holistic health, mankind can have an uplift. All he has to do is make the decision, each for himself. Whatever you choose for yourself is right. With that decision comes an uplift. It could be physical, mental, and spiritual.

The physical uplift can be seen in many ways, from the lifting of the bosom to an actual increase in body height. The mental directions of head rising are "uplift" from the word go. Many students describe this as also a spiritual experience.

Combining more than one method would bring about an even greater "uplift" of the whole person. Some Alexander teachers have two or more careers, and they share them both with their students and clients.

A physiotherapist in New York is also an Alexander teacher. It is a happy "marriage." Deborah Caplan is a Director of the American Center for the Alexander Technique, Inc. in New York. She gets referrals from medical people in the area of physiotherapy. Physiotherapists often give their patients corrective exercises, and often the patient is unable to do them either because too much pain already exists, or because pain is caused by these exercises.

What these therapists do not consider or understand is that exercises can be done with or without strain. Caplan understands this and teaches her Alexander students to go through therapeutic exercises in a stressless way so that they enjoy the therapeutic benefits without pain. Naturally, they also get the benefits of Alexander lessons with her.

Another Alexander teacher I know was also a dance teacher, in Tel Aviv, Israel. Her name is Katya Michaeli. Her dance students all had Alexander lessons, as a separate part of her program. During the dance classes, she moved around, touching her students lightly, reminding them of their Alexander directions. A student of mine in New York, a former ballerina, went to Michaeli for lessons when she visited Israel. She reported to me that what beginners were doing in Michaeli's initial movement classes was beyond what even some advanced dancers were able to do with other teachers.

Virginia Wagner used to teach both Alexander and T'ai chi in Los Angeles, recommending that her T'ai chi students take Alexander lessons. Her experience had shown that T'ai chi students made faster progress when they had reeducated the daily use of their bodies. Similarly, she frequently recommended T'ai chi movements for certain Alexander students.

There are Alexander teachers who also teach physiosynthesis, the Laban Method, and other approaches. The majority of Alexander teachers who teach other approaches as well as Alexander, usually do not combine the two together, but rather offer one as a supplement to or reinforcement for the other. A student who goes to one of these teachers for Alexander lessons is likely to get pure Alexander lessons, as well as the possibility of adding another approach. Any Alexander teacher who is familiar with other helpful methods can enhance the Alexander lessons with their additional knowledge.

I myself have been teaching the Feldenkrais method of Awareness through Movement for several years, in addition to my Alexander teaching.

Feldenkrais' exercise-like movements, like Alexander, are done not with a desire to reach a goal, but with an awareness of *how* we move.

Some of my Alexander students came to my Feldenkrais classes, which are group sessions, and some Feldenkrais students come for Alexander. When this happens, I see an obvious acceleration in the student's progress.

It helps me, too. My additional understanding of how the body moves through Feldenkrais has enhanced my Alexander skills. I am able to assist students of mine who do exercises prescribed by physiotherapists and orthopedists by teaching them the Feldenkrais approach to movement; I am also able to achieve Alexander break-throughs for certain students by teaching them special Feldenkrais movements—circumventing pain and improving limberness—as as adjunct to the Alexander Technique.

Two other Alexander teachers that I know teach the Feldenkrais Method in addition to the Alexander Technique. Frank Ottiwell, who is the resident Alexander teacher with the American Conservatory Theater in San Francisco, teaches the company Feldenkrais and Alexander with great success, as can be seen by the way the company moves on stage. Ilana Rubenfeld of New York City started her career as a choral conductor, became an Alexander teacher, and in addition has since become a Gestalt Therapist and Feldenkrais teacher.

Paul Gleason of Hollywood became an Alexander teacher while continuing a long-standing career of teaching acting and dance. He is currently Associate Director of the Civic Light Opera Musical Theatre Workshop at the Music Center in Los Angeles, and combines this career with Alexander teaching.

There are others who have become Alexander teachers who are psychologists, voice teachers, drama teachers, piano teachers, yoga, and dance teachers.

Self-Improvement Doors That Open

People who take Alexander lessons often find a new world of interests. Some are ordinary nine-to-five job holders with no outside interests apart from paying off the mortgage. Then, when they take Alexander lessons, for some reason these interests expand. They might go to a gym, or start a continuing education course, or take up a sport, a foreign language, a musical instrument, or meditation.

A middle-aged couple who had never done any mind-body techniques, consciousness expansion, therapy, or human potential training signed up for Alexander lessons. They were a conventional suburban couple with grown children. First she came for lessons because of great pain. Her crabbiness disappeared with her pains and she became witty and delightful. Then her husband also came for lessons, complaining of a pain in the neck, which I might conjecture was originally caused by his reaction to her crabbiness. He, too, experienced a relief from pain and a personality change. His manner turned from gruff and negative to humorous and caring.

When they were both taking Alexander lessons they found it was a medium for greater closeness to each other. They then began to investigate other mind-body approaches. They took workshops at Esalen Institute. They enrolled for massage workshops. Next, they got themselves a hot tub, the first in their neighborhood to have a large redwood tub with a jacuzzi jet in it. She wrote an article for *Wet* magazine on whether a middle-aged couple could find happiness with a hot tub. She went on to write humorous articles for other magazines.

They have gone on to become interested in Gestalt Therapy, bio-energetics, Rajneesh meditations, and other approaches to a fuller life. They are today more open to new approaches than are their children.

They are a popular couple. They meet a far broader spectrum of people, and are found to be charming and delightful by those whom they meet.

I myself experienced an expansion in my thinking as my body became more open. I used to avoid thinking in philosophical terms. I was quite cynical about metaphysical and spiritual theories, and now I find I have a more open and thoughtful attitude toward these matters. Whereas such subjects as ESP and reincarnation used to send me scurrying, today I am happy to discuss them. Negativity in my body reflected in negativity in my philosophy of life. The downward droop of my body has been replaced by an upward lift and a corresponding upward lift has taken place in my philosophical concepts.

Formerly, I could not care less where we all came from or where we were all going. Now, not only do I take an interest, but I feel a oneness with those ideas. Also, my intuitive perceptions seem to be on the increase. My body is part of it. If I hear somebody say something, I might feel my body contract slightly. It is a signal to me that the answer to that is no, it is not a good thing. Other times what is said will induce a feeling of expansion. I will feel my body lengthening and widening. That is my intuitive signal that it is a good thing. I feel similar signals when meeting people: I have an immediate reaction that is a combination of perception and an inner sensation that I experience as a contraction or expansion. The differences are subtle, but through the subtlety of the Alexander Technique I can now recognize other subtleties.

➡ The Dance of Life

Many Alexander students say that, for the first time in their lives, they are enjoying dancing. They say that people remark admiringly about them, that their bodies move in new and exciting ways. Some say that now, whenever there is music, they can hardly contain themselves. They must get up and move to the music, expressing themselves to music, something they had never done before. Some start doing this alone, others do it unabashedly at parties. The admiration of others feeds their confidence in their newfound self.

It is typical of an office worker to tell me that now he enjoys the feeling of his body so much, he frequently gets up from his desk to walk up and down the office or corridor.

All kinds of tasks and mundane activities which were boring chores now feel like dance-like activities. The words some people use in describing this cannot help but remind me of descriptions of the lightness and buoyancy that our astronauts brought back from the moon.

John Dewey has described how he was a person who had wanted to get through the physical activities of his life as quickly as possible, and get on with the mental work. He wrote of this in one of the prefaces he wrote for three of Alexander's books. He went on to explain that through the Alexander Technique he discovered that there was a whole way of life involved in his physical activities that changed his attitude toward his work and his life. He also gained the benefit of changing ill health to good health. He was 56, and in ill health, when he went to Alexander, and he gives credit to the Alexander work for his ensuing good health. Dewey lived to be over 90 years of age.

Dewey made a strong effort to interest foundations and universities in sponsoring research into the Technique. He had great confidence in the Technique, "having living proof in myself," but he became resigned to the likelihood that its recognition by the academic world must wait.

That time has now arrived, and we see the first steps of an interest in academia in the Alexander Technique as a freeing of the mind for superior learning. So far it has been confined to Departments of Music, Drama, Dance and Biological and Physical Sciences. This is only the beginning. It is clear that the trend will spread.

Individuals in every walk of life are becoming aware of this alternative through education by the mass media. These individuals are experiencing an awakening through the Alexander Technique. Its manifestation can come in a desire to dance more or it can come in making all life a joyous dance.

In the Alexander Technique we learn not only how to be in that joyous place, but also when we feel we are slipping back a little bit, we have a way to bring ourselves out of it through our mental directions. Once you know how it is to feel joyous, once you know what it is like to feel light and delicious, then anything less than that is not satisfactory.

This is corroborated in an article called "Getting Your Back Straight" by Jeanne du Prau, which appeared in *New Realities*, Vol. 1, No. 5. The author explains that she went for Alexander lessons because of a painful back resulting from a scoliosis. She had failed to have success with medically prescribed methods, and wished to avoid surgery. She suffered from stiff necks and cricks in the back, in addition to pain and inability to sit comfortably. After four months of lessons, she had no stiff necks or cricks in the back, could sit comfortably, quite straight, for an hour or more, and goes on to say:

"I don't want to sound like one of those unpleasant people who has found the One True Path to health, happiness, and inner peace . . . but the Alexander Technique makes a radical change in those who practice it: it takes you off the road to disintegration and sets you on the road to improvement instead. . . .

"Now, instead of dismally noting the symptoms of my decay, I count the signs of progress. I feel strong where I used to feel weak, relaxed where I used to feel tense, I look better to other people . . . I am less depressed, irritable, and tired . . . I have acquired a new vision of my future. I am not going to be the grouchy and decrepit oldster I began feeling like last year. I will be instead one of those people who becomes both calmer and more energetic with the passage of time. Fifty years from now, when my contemporaries are stooped and slow, I will be a strong, erect old lady."

➡️ Effortless Living

You can float through life.

Everything you do can be as if you were riding on "cloud nine."

Wherever you go, traveling by foot, bicycle, or car can be effortless. Whoever you meet or deal with can be a pleasurable, harmonious experience. It comes about from reversing the effort process through Alexander instructions.

By "seeing" your head go forward and up in gentle movements, you are freeing your body and mind from the weight that is continuously making demands on you for your effort.

It works so universally that I do not say to you, you must do it five times a day or ten times a day or fifteen times a day. I do not say to you, repeat the directions for one minute or three minutes. I do not say to you that you should select a particular activity like walking, or sitting, or standing, or lifting, as the movement with which to give the directions.

All I can say is: give them. Give the directions daily, not only when you feel tension or stress, but at any time.

Your life will be uplifted. Your life will be effortless.

The ease and gentleness of the Alexander Technique can permeate all experiences. Life can become serene, peaceful, and more interesting as you discover more about yourself and others through your newly developed awareness. Relationships with others can become more loving and understanding, and often more exciting as you develop more aliveness.

With science's new discoveries about brain waves, it becomes easier to understand why we affect other people in ways that vary with our moods and consciousness. Your "vibes" are picked up at a subliminal level. It has been said that 99 percent of all environmental input to the body and mind is at a subliminal or unconscious level.

Somebody may not be aware of why he opposes your wish, goal or idea, but he takes an opposing stand nevertheless. Below the level of consciousness, signals are being received, "This is an uptight person, disordered, disconnected, and pressured. No rapport is invited."

Good body use brings a more tranquil mind. Signals from such a mind are quite different, "This is an 'in-tune' person, ordered like the Universe, connected to its Source, and in balance with the times. Rapport can be of optimum benefit."

The buyer buys from you. The lover loves you. The judge dismisses the charges against you.

Something else happens.

Once you have done the Alexander experiences and the exercises in this book to make you more body-aware, once you have given yourself Alexander directions repeatedly for postural improvement and improved use of your body, any reversion to your old self becomes an aversion.

You are instantly aware of your slumpy body or grumpy mind because it has a bad feeling and you instantly change it. Giving yourself the Alexander directions at such a moment is part of the undoing process.

Some years ago *Newsweek* wanted to write an article on the Alexander Technique. They asked if I would come to their studio and demonstrate good and poor use for the photographers.

After demonstrating good use, I repeated over and over poor use in sitting, standing, and walking. To do this I reverted to the old habits I had had before taking Alexander lessons—the sway back that used to give me backaches, the slumping down, and added other common bad habits. By the time I was ready to go home, I was feeling terrible. I was feeling as I did in the days when I thought life wasn't worth living. My jaw hung open and I felt like a dribbling idiot.

It took some doing for me to pull out of that and get back to good use.

You risk the same regression by pemitting yourself to reinforce poor use, by permitting yourself to continue in the same old way.

Instead, when you sit, stand, or walk, give yourself Alexander directions. Give the directions many times. Feel the uplift. Good use needs the reinforcement of daily remembrance of mental directions.

Did you know that the billions of neurons in your brain have a natural tendency to seek pleasure and avoid pain? That is what the theory of A. Harry Klopf, who did his research at the Air Force Avionics Laboratory at Wright-Patterson Air Force Base in Ohio, seems to point to. Neurons are hedonists, he believes, constantly seeking excitation and pleasure. Klopf finds that the brain can no longer be seen as a collection of logic units, but rather as ''an organized population of billions of goal-seeking 'creatures' each 'talking' to some thousands of others and each adapting in behavior in accordance with whether or not it is getting what it wants.''*

Your brain votes for joy.

It will make toting that barge and lifting that bale effortless, and your body and mind can sing about it. Joy and new joyful experiences are what life is all about.

We are not meant to suffer. Nature has endowed us with oxygen as the breath of life and joy as its nourishment.

➡ Be Kind to Yourself: Tips I Give My Alexander Students

Here are some of the helpful hints I tell my Alexander students that contribute to a way of life that goes hand-in-hand with our Alexander learning. Many of the students discover these ways for themselves as a by-product of their Alexander lessons, others need to be shown the way.

BE KIND TO YOURSELF, MOVE GENTLY. Notice when you feel that you are rushing, straining, or working hard compulsively. When you drive your car, are you strenuously gripping the steering wheel? You actually can control your car more efficiently with a light

*Brain-Mind Bulletin, May 1, 1978, P.O. Box 42211, Los Angeles, CA 90042.

touch. Your reflexes can come through faster when you have a light touch. And so it is with everything you do. When you walk, are you rushing? Slow down, walk gently, and *enjoy* your walk. When you sit down on a chair, sit down gently; instead of landing on the chair with a thump, come down airily and meet the chair softly. When you stand up, come up *gently*. When carrying a shopping bag, or attaché case, do you feel that you are gripping it very hard? You can carry it just as easily with less work. When pulling out drawers, are you exerting a lot of muscle power, so that you pull hard on a drawer that slides out easily? Instead, you could do it with a light touch of the fingers. And so on through all the movements of your daily life. Become aware, if you can, of the extra work you do and, once you are aware of it, you can eliminate at least some of it by moving more gently; and you can eliminate more by giving Alexander directions. That is being kind to yourself.

You can be kinder to other people by touching gently. When you shake a person's hand, are you gripping them so hard that their bones crunch? I am not suggesting that your hand be floppy, just eliminate some of the extra work. When you stroke someone, when you massage someone, when you pat someone on the back, are you putting unnecessary additional work into it? Do it gently. *Treat others as gently as you would like to be treated yourself.*

AVOID EXHAUSTION. Another way to be kind to yourself is to pace yourself gently, and to take frequent rest breaks. It makes a great difference to both the quantity and quality of what you can accomplish when you take time out every so often, instead of driving yourself to exhaustion. Your rest breaks do not need to be long when they are frequent—just short periods of time out from whatever you are doing, whether it be physical activity or mental activity. It can also be very helpful when you are in an emotional bind.

A rest break can mean different things: you could take a complete physical rest and lie down on the floor with your knees bent, and, if you wish, "Alexander" yourself; or, if you are not involved in an activity that is physically straining to your whole body, you may wish to take a break by doing something different, and then returning to your original activity. Scientific experiments have shown that muscles can have fully functioning energy over a long period of time when given frequent rest breaks, whereas a muscle that is given no rest becomes weaker and weaker and eventually is totally inactive. This applies to our minds, emotions and bodies. You can apply the principle of rest breaks to all areas of your life. *Become more aware of yourself, and through that, be good to yourself.*

STAY WARM. This is also being kind to yourself. When you are cold your muscles tighten and contract. By staying warm, you prevent the tightening and excessive contraction, and you can remain lengthened. Wear warm clothing. Do not be heroic when it is cold and chilly, and say, "Oh, I'm warm enough." Do not leave windows wide open when the weather is cold. I am an advocate of fresh air, and I am not asking you to close your windows completely and make your room stuffy, but just enough to keep the room warm. Or, if you like your windows wide open in cold weather, dress more warmly. In cold weather, I recommend that my students wear an extra sweater, a pair of stockings or long johns, or panty hose or leotards under their slacks, or to wear thermal underwear. You will be far more comfortable when you are warm and your whole organism will thank you for it.

WARM BATHS AND SAUNAS. Warm baths, saunas, and soaking in hot jacuzzi pools are very therapeutic for the muscles and are almost like a treatment that allows your body to become softer, more gentle, and less contracted. Then, when you give your Alexander thoughts, your body can flow more readily into the lengthening and widening direction.

Please *do not overdo saunas and hot pools.* A good recommendation is that as soon as you start sweating, get out and take a cold shower, or a dip in a cold pool. Then you can return to the sauna or hot tub, and when you start sweating again, get out and take another cold shower or cold dip. This way you can get the full benefit of the heat without becoming listless and drowsy. You will retain your energy and feel refreshed and invigorated, as well as relaxed. If it is late at night, and you want to go to sleep afterwards, it is not a good idea to invigorate yourself; at such times, I recommend a lukewarm shower following a sauna or a hot tub, and you will be in a very relaxed state, ready to go to sleep.

WEAR COMFORTABLE CLOTHING. Another way to be

good to yourself. When you wear tight clothing, muscles contract. Sometimes you may not be aware of it immediately; you may be feeling uncomfortable and not know why; later, you take off your tight clothing and you breathe a sigh of relief, and say, "Oh, I feel much more comfortable now"; and your breathing is also freer. Your sigh of relief was the release of your breath that was constricted as a result of the tight clothing. See that your belt and the crotch of your pants are not too tight, that blouses are not too snug, that the shoulders of shirts and blouses are not too narrow, that collars and hats are not too confining. Most comfortable of all, of course, is loose clothing. Sometimes, though, we want to wear snug-fitting clothes that look elegant, or show off our figures. *Be aware of the difference between snug-fitting clothing and tight clothing.*.

SHOES ARE VERY IMPORTANT. Wear shoes and sandals with comfortable soles. Rigid soles do not allow your feet to move freely and the muscles and joints can become stiff. For flexible feet, wear flexible shoes.

HIGH-HEELED SHOES ARE EXTREMELY HARMFUL TO THE BACK, THE CALF MUSCLES, AND THE ACHILLES TENDON. Backaches can develop from wearing high heels, in addition to tension in the legs and tightness in the hip joints. High heels usually throw the back out of alignment. Those of us who already have weak muscles in the back are endangering our backs by wearing anything but low heels or flat heels.

Any of you who have worn high heels constantly probably find that when you wear flat heels it makes your calf muscles sore. That is because those muscles have become shortened from wearing high heels, and when wearing flat heels you are stretching those muscles beyond what they have become accustomed to. You may get discouraged and say, "I'm much more comfortable in high heels." What I recommend is that you *gradually wean yourself away from high heels.*

Wear flat heels perhaps for half an hour at first, then for an hour a day, then two hours and three hours. When you wean yourself gradually from high heels, you can avoid the pain; you will be *gradually* stretching out and lengthening the muscles of your calves and your tendons, until eventually that will feel normal to you. The next time you put on high heels, when you are no longer used to them, you will feel how uncomfortable your legs are, and you may also feel what it is doing to your back.

GET ENOUGH SLEEP. Be good to yourself, and sleep a full night's sleep. When you do not sleep enough, your muscles tighten. Every movement you do during the day with tight muscles is causing more strain, more difficulty, and the muscles tighten even more from the strain, and it becomes a vicious cycle. You can prevent this by sleeping the number of hours that is adequate for you; for most people it is six, seven, or eight hours. I have met people who say they have trained themselves to sleep fewer hours, maybe four or five hours a night. When I looked at these people, I saw that their bodies were tense, their muscles were tight, and they were not moving smoothly and easily.

It is up to you to find out how much sleep is enough for you. For myself, the degree of sleep that I need varies. I need more sleep when I am working, I need less sleep when I am on vacation. When I work part-time, I need something in between.

Be aware of what feels like adequate sleep for you, and do not take what is adequate for one night as the rule for every night of your life. You need to be aware of how much energy you are putting out during the day, and adjust your sleep accordingly. This, among other things that I ask of you, is a matter of developing your self-awareness. When you sleep, choose a position that is the most comfortable for your body, a position that does not keep you in a tight contracted position all night.

Alexander students experience that when they lack sleep, they lose some of their good direction and some of the lovely benefits that come with it; however, after they have rested well, the good direction returns. On days when you feel more rigid, stiffer and heavier in your body, ask yourself whether you had enough sleep the previous night, or nights. If the answer is no, make time for a nap to restore the elasticity to your muscles and the vibrant tone to your body. A note of warning: the loss of elasticity in muscles from lack of sleep can become permanent, or semi-permanent, when lack of sufficient sleep has continued over a period of weeks or longer.

SWIM. Swimming is one of the most highly recommended sports for exercise. The reason is that you are supported by the water. When the water supports you, you put far less effort into the movements than you would if you did the same movements while standing upright and having to support yourself against gravity. This does not mean that everyone swims without overexerting them-selves. What it means is that they exert themselves *less* than they would if they did movements while being vertical: there is some elimination of overwork in movements done in the water.

Swimmers usually have long, smooth muscles, not bulging or knotted, nor tight and stringy. Runners tend to have long stringy muscles; weight lifters tend to have hard bunched muscles. I think swimming is the form of exercise that is much more likely to give you the long, smooth musculature that is the most efficient for good use. Such muscles have good tone and are elastic. Muscles that are tight and stringy can tear easily, as they are not elastic enough, and the same can happen with muscles that are bunched and hard.

I once had a conversation with a "muscle man" who was runner-up that year in the Mr. Universe contest. He told me that he did not do any physical activity outside of walking slowly and the exercises prescribed for his muscle building. He never walked fast, he never ran, he never went into the water and swam. The reason he gave was that he would hurt his muscles. He was an extreme example of what happens when you are muscle-bound. Those hard, bulging muscles tear very easily. Perhaps, if he had taken Alexander lessons, he would have learned how to move in other activities without tearing muscles. Tearing muscles is much more unlikely with swimmers.

There is a way of making your swimming easier, less tiring, and more beneficial. Give your Alexander directions. As you are swim-ming, think of the top of your head going out ahead of you and think of your neck and back lengthening, following your head; *do not try and push yourself into length*, merely give the command mentally. If you want to use only one thought, *use the thought of lengthening*. I think you will find swimming quite different.

BREATHE. Do not hold your breath. *All you need to do to breathe well is to be aware of your breathing*. Simply notice your breathing. Please do not try to do anything exaggerated with your breathing. I am referring to breathing in your daily life, not to breathing exercises. I am suggesting that every so often you simply notice your breath; as soon as you notice your breath, you will be breathing normally and well without having to try, without doing anything special about it. As soon as you notice your breath, you may find that you have been holding your breath, and all of a sudden the breath flows easily and smoothly. Breathing is as easy as that.

When you are going to do something that takes more effort, more energy and exertion, then intentionally *reathe out*. Let us say you have to push a table across the room. Just before you push it, inhale so that you can exhale while you push the table. When you are doing any kind of exercises, *exhale as you do the active part of the exercise*, and inhale as you release it. In our culture, we seem to have been taught just the opposite, either by direct teaching, or by an attitude. We mostly hold our breath when we are about to do something. Holding the breath is something we do when we are frightened, and we also hold our breath when we are anxious. See what it feels like to inhale and hold your breath. Can you feel the muscles in the back and sides of your neck tighten, and also your shoulders, and can you feel your chest become stiff and your belly become rigid? Just imagine how difficult it is to do an exercise or exertive movement when your muscles are in that state. Now let go of your breath. Do you feel the softness and ease in your whole body as a result of your muscles having released their tension?

Muscles move much more easily on the exhalation, and you will find that any exercises that you do will be far easier, more pleasurable, and bring about greater suppleness when you do them on the exhalation. Any activity that you do that requires a little more effort than normal will become much easier when you exhale. Many people hurt themselves when they do exercises while inhaling, and when they do something like pushing a table while inhaling. They hurt their backs or strain a muscle, or go into muscle spasm; a lot of this can be avoided by breathing out instead of breathing in at such times.

DO NOT TWIST YOUR SPINE. I would like you to think of your torso as one unit. Your torso is the part of your body that goes from your hip joints and your tailbone all the way to the top of your neck. Your limbs, which are your two legs and your two arms, are attached to the torso, and your head is attached onto the top of your spine. The head is often called, half-jokingly, the "fifth limb." There is no part of your spine that has a major joint in it to allow it to twist around easily, or bend easily. There is no joint in your back like the joint in your elbow or the joint in your wrist, shoulder or knee. Your limbs can bend backwards easily because of the joints, and also because the muscles around them are long muscles that stretch easily, like long elastic bands. In your back, although you have long muscles, you also have short muscles, The short muscles do not stretch easily. They have a limited elasticity and that is why they protest when they are constantly used incorrectly and have been forced to stretch more than is appropriate.

To open a drawer, stand in front of the drawer and face it, rather that standing to one side and twisting around. When laying carpet in your bathroom, let's say, see that you do not twist around into strange contortions. Instead, turn your whole body around so that you are always facing the part you are working on and not twisting around.

Here is another area where *I am asking you to be aware, and to be kind to yourself*. You can avoid back pain and strained muscles simply by using good common sense. That is really what this is all about—good common sense. When you are kind to yourself, and good to yourself, you will be so much more comfortable with yourself that you can be kinder to others, and do more good to those around you.

AVOID BENDING BACKWARDS. There are some people whose back muscles are so limber that they can do backbends with the greatest of ease, and not hurt themselves. But are you one of those people? Probably not, or you would not be reading this book. The majority of us do not have such flexible backs. The muscles of our backs are not designed to bend backwards, so it is a difficult movement for them. It is over-stretching them in a direction in which they are not designed to go, and it squeezes the vertebrae together. People who have extreme flexibility can do this without hurting themselves. One can be trained to achieve that flexibility, although some people are not in good enough condition to ever be able to do it.

In daily life, avoid bending backwards.

If you are doing Yoga, or any exercises where you do some

movements that bend you backwards, think of lengthening while
you do it, and immediately afterwards do some gentle movements
that will counteract the effects of the backbend, movements that will
move your body in the opposite direction.

I would like to show you a movement that I have found to be one of
the most successful. There are many movements one can do to bring
relief to the muscles after a backbend, and this is one of them.

Lie down on the floor and gently draw your legs up one at a time,
legs and feet apart. Clasp your hands behind your head. *Very gently*,
lift your arms and head off the floor, a little bit, and lift your right foot

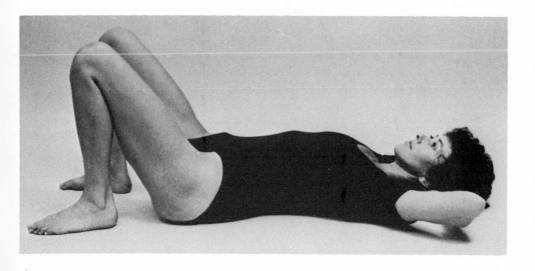

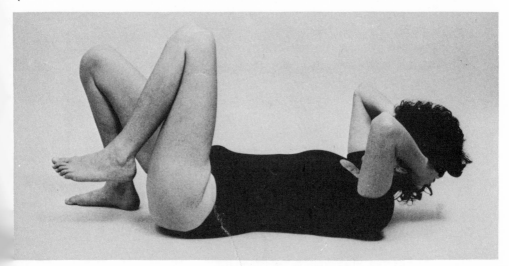

a little bit, and lower them all to the floor. Do *not* hold yourself in the air. Do this a few times, slowly and easily. Now do a few movements with the left foot. *Do the movement as you exhale softly through your mouth.*

Many people tend to do big movements. They try to get the elbow and knee to touch or to get them very close to each other. That is not the point of this movement. To satisfy your urge to get them to touch, the next time you do this movement, try and get your elbow and knee to touch, and go back again. From now on, I would like you to *do one-third of that movement.* Go only one-third of the way, and do the movement in this small gentle way. Maybe five or six times. It is a gentle movement that has to do with moving the flexor muscles of your torso, and releasing the extensor muscles in your back. *The movement is much easier when you do it on your exhalation.* When your head is on the floor, inhale lightly, gently, and when you lift your arms and foot, exhale slowly and softly through your mouth.

While you do the movement, notice what goes on in your back. Which part of your back is coming up off the floor? And which part of your back is being pressed against the floor?

Now come to resting. Gently take your hands out from behind your head, lower your arms to your sides and lower your legs one at a time. While resting, think of how your body is lying on the floor. Do you feel any difference in your back, and in other parts of your body?

You can do variations of this movement. You can do it alternating

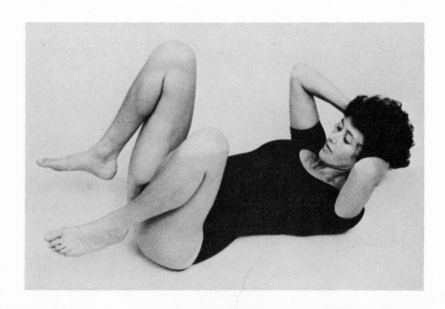

left foot and right foot, and you can do it lifting both feet at the same time as lifting your head and arms. If you are eager to do all the variations, give yourself a rest break on the floor after you have done five or six movements. Wait for at least three breaths to pass before you continue.

You can bring more pleasure into your life, not only through directing your "uplift" through "neck free, head forward and up, back lengthening and widening," but also by choosing pleasurable ways of going through your daily life. The choice is yours between stress and joy. At first, you need to be consciously aware of the difference in your various activities, then *gradually your body will automatically choose the pleasurable way*.

➡ How to Get More Benefit From Exercises

You can use Alexander directions to help you with calisthenics or limbering-up exercises.

There are certain things that exercises cannot do. Rarely do they improve posture or good body use. If a person has hunched shoulders and a tight back, he does exercises with shoulders hunched and back tight. This merely reinforces the poor use, and it can even do harm.

Even in physiotherapy, the patients walk out of the session with the same posture they had when they walked in, by admission of the therapists themselves who admit it is a "long pull."

This need not be so. You can use your Alexander instructions in physiotherapy or in your "daily dozen" and convert them from a reinforcer of poor habits—low levels of well-being—to the reinforcer of good habits, leading to higher and higher levels of joyous well-being.

In the process, you will also find that the exercises will be more fun. You will realize how much strain, effort, and discomfort you have been experiencing while doing the exercises. Now, with good posture and better use of your body in the exercises, you will be getting the maximum benefit from them with the least effort.

Let us take the knee-bend. You place your hands on your hips, or you have your arms in front of you, and you lower yourself by

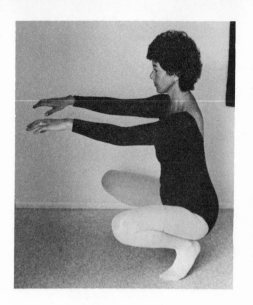
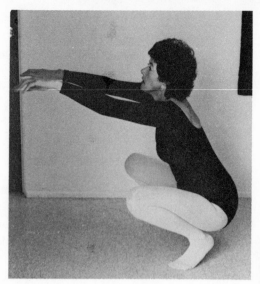

bending your knees, then raise yourself by straightening your knees. One, two, one, two. If you wish to do this, do it three or four times in the way you would normally do it.

Now review this familiar exercise mentally, adding your Alexander directions. Mentally, place your hands on your hips or bring your arms in front of you, mentally lower your chin slightly and give yourself the directions: "Neck free, head forward and up, back lengthening and widening"; mentally do the exercise while continuing to think the directions. Do it in your mind about three times.

Now actually do it, *slowly and gently*, as you continue to say the Alexander thoughts to yourself. You need not think of step one, bending the knees, or step two, straightening them. You already know what you are to do. You can do the movements without thinking of them, and your mind is free to dwell on the mental directions. Repeat them over and over, as you bend and straighten. This is probably a different experience for you than before. Do you find the movement easier, lighter?

When you do exercises with good use, and with ease and gentleness, you will find in the long run that you are getting as much benefit, and probably more, without needing to do as many exercises, or as often. The exercises can become less enervating, more stimulating, *and* more pleasurable, so that you will actually enjoy doing your exercises.

Exercising does not change your habits. It does increase your circulation and benefit your body cells, but it will not correct a mother's back alignment that went wrong from carrying a baby, or an office worker's back alignment from slumping over a desk.

However, if you couple your exercises with your Alexander directions, yours is the best of both worlds; a toned-up, limber body, and the reinforcement of good body habits.

Alexander students who do a routine program of exercises are finding that the exercises are now doing for them what they were supposed to do, but did not do before. Doing the exercises with good use of the body is bringing about the effects that the exercises were designed for.

Other Alexander students discontinue their exercises, as they find that the Alexander Technique is doing for them what the exercises were supposed to have done and did not do. Their muscles are strengthened and their bodies reproportioned.

My observation is that Alexander students who are doing a reasonable amount of physical activity in their daily lives, such as walking to and from work, to and from the bus, or to and from shopping, have not needed exercises to keep their bodies in good shape.

However, those who lead a very sedentary life do need to do some activity, whether it be exercises or exercise. Without activity, the body does become stiffer, and flabbier. Good use of the muscles and the body can take care of a myriad troubles, but *one must use the body to employ the good use.*

I have often met friends whom I have not seen for many years. Some of them look heavier to me, particularly around the midriff and hips. They tell me that they have not gained weight over the years, but their bodies have changed—for the worse. Some of them say despairingly that they go faithfully to the gym and exercise there, and, although they feel good afterwards, it does not make any difference to their figures. They look at me and remark that my body has gone in the opposite direction, that I look better than when I was younger: "You must exercise a lot," they say. "No, I do no real exercise, and no sports," I reply, "it's Alexander." And so say many other "Alexandrians."

My own experience has been that while I lived in New York,

where I walked frequently, Alexander lessons smoothed and firmed my flabby thighs and buttocks, and toned and reproportioned my body beautifully. After moving to California, where I rely on my car for transportation and do not give time to swimming or other exercise, my flabbiness started to return, and my back was starting to lose some of its limberness. To take care of myself, I do some gentle Feldenkrais movements for about five minutes most mornings to keep my body limber and supple.

I have found that whenever I am walking more, as I do when on vacation, I have no need to supplement the daily activities of my life. Walking, sitting, standing and bending with good use is the best toning of the body that I, and many others, have found.

▶ Unveiling a Joyous You

Through familiarity, and habit, you had become comfortable with a body that was bent and tightened by the ravages of a stressful world, but once you experience the new lightness that the movements and mental directions provided on these pages can bring, you are likely to be satisfied with nothing else.

This is the true unveiling of a new you.

You have been exhilarated in the past by a cold shower, a swim in the ocean or pool, a workout in the gym. But, it has been temporary. You enjoyed it while it lasted, knowing that the buoyancy would pass.

Now you know a different exhilaration. It is a lightness that is the real "you" returning. Yes, you feel like a new person after a swim or a workout, but what you feel after restoring good use through giving yourself mental directions over a period of time, is the former "you." It is the "you" you once knew before you developed the tense neck, crooked legs, sway back, pained back, aches, and pains.

You are unveiling the joyous child that you once were before you developed the layers of armoring, ego-protection, and scar tissue from life's punches.

The real, joyous you has been there right along.

Do not make the mistake of thinking that the lightness is just of the body. The same brain that causes the lightness of the body is interpreting the impulses being received as sights, sounds, tastes, smells, and touches. I promise you that you will see another person differently and that person will be picking up an alternate impression of you.

A handsome young actor who comes for Alexander lessons used to have a rigid, nonhandsome body. His stiff swayed back, protruding butt, collapsed chest and shoulders shouted anything but "Hollywood," and he was the first to admit it. As heavy as his body was when I worked with him at first, that is how light it feels now. His posture is realigned.

And also "realigned" is his outlook on life. His chest is broader and so are his interests. His shoulders are stronger, and so is his character. His face now radiates, as does his personality.

This is growth. This young man said to me one day, "Girls that looked good to me in my pre-Alexander days don't interest me today. Most girls I look at today, whom I would have dated at the drop of an eyelid in the past, are unappealing to me nowadays because of their poor bodies. I never saw them that way before. Now, when I see someone with a long smooth line in their body, I admire it and want to know that person."

When we begin to feel ourselves in a better place, it is natural for us to feel the need for people who are not where we used to be, but who are also in this better place.

We are lighter. We rise to a higher level. We acquire, require, and attract a higher level of consciousness. This leads to a higher level of wealth—wealth of experience, of possessions, and of joyous relationships with other joyous people.

➡ How To Be Successful At Being Selfish

Happy. Delicious. Joyous. Buoyant.

Once you attain this body-mind euphoria, you will do anything to protect it and maintain it.

That is how the healing arts started in ancient times. The need to take something for a physical discomfort so as to restore well-being led to the evolution of the medicine man and eventually to the physician.

You can now use mental directions like medicine to maintain your euphoric well-being. This maintenance of well-being becomes so important that it is a part of your very philosophy of life. Having once known what misdirection can do to your body and mind, you become dedicated to good direction in order to have a firm foundation to face life.

You know that life can blast you with bombardment after bombardment of stressful circumstances which can cripple you, dull your mental acumen, and lower your stature among your peers.

No more.

Your head is up. Your back is erect. Your future is secure. You attract able, confident, secure people into your life. They feel they can relate to you, and you feel you can relate to them.

Each of you affects the other. You will see some of your friends, who have not taken Alexander lessons or done the substitute lessons in this book, begin to have better posture from being around you. They will pick it up by "osmosis." They will not necessarily know that they are standing straighter, but they will know that for some reason they enjoy being with you. They feel uplifted by your presence.

Your ease and vitality will also be sensed and subconsciously emulated. More and more people in your business, social, and family circles will feel more warm and open.

Your selfish concern for your own body-mind well-being will, in this way, radiate to others. You will be giving benefit to others by being selfish. How much better you and I will be if more people were selfish in this way. We will be making this a better world to live in.

▶ How You Can Help Others In Pain

You help others with whom you come in contact simply by being your more joyous, buoyant self. There is also specific help that you can give to family, friends, and co-workers who are in pain.

These people are often on medication to relieve the pain of arthritis, rheumatism, bursitis, and backache. When on medication, these people are not fully alert. They are half-drugged. They are going through life in less than a vital way.

Most of these people who come for Alexander lessons find that their pain is either partially or totally relieved after a few lessons and eventually can be a thing of the past. They can stop the drugged life and resume an alert life.

How do you fit into this picture? If you know such a person, you have, through the means by which you helped yourself with this book, the means to help others.

The mini-Alexander lesson on page 172 is your best starting point. You can either refer the person in pain to this procedure or you can read the directions to him.

There is no danger in lying down on a well-padded floor or table, with a book or two under your head. Bending the knees with the feet flat on the floor is a natural position, not an exercise. Some may need to have their knees propped up with pillows.

Going through this mini-Alexander lesson for a few minutes, with all mental directions as spelled out, will begin a reversal of many muscle-bone pains.

Sometimes it is difficult to have someone in pain to agree to even this simple, natural "nondoing" movement. They have little regard for the mind's role in their pain problem, and why risk more pain with no promise of relief?

Here is a simple way to "break the ice." If somebody has a pain, tell them you have a mental way to help them get rid of it. Tell them that all they need to do is answer your questions.

Then you follow this line of questioning.

1. Ask them to point to exactly where the pain is located.
2. Ask them, "If this pain could fit in a container, what kind of a container would you need to put it in?"
3. Ask them, "If this pain had a color, what color would it be?" Insist on an answer, even if they have to make it up.
4. Ask them, "If this pain had a taste, what would it taste like?" Again, insist on a conscientious attempt to assign a taste.
5. Ask them, "If this pain had a smell, what would it smell like?" Again, insist on an answer, any smell that comes to mind.
6. Ask them again to point to the pain.

If the pain still exists, go through the other five steps of this cycle again. Usually, after three rounds, even a migraine headache can be largely relieved.

Once you have effected an improvement, clinch your point.

"See how the mind can affect pain? Now, shall we take the next step?"

Your friend will probably be convinced and you can go on to share what you know about the Alexander Technique by reading the mini-lesson and having the person give himself the mental directions that could begin to undo the cause of the pain. You would be getting a person that is lost to this world by dint of pain-killing drugs back into full awareness and enjoyment of life.

There is a leaning on the part of scientists today to look upon the universe with emphasis on the "uni." A continuum concept has replaced the "nothingness" concept. Space is "somethingness" with properties. One of these properties appears to be the transmittal of thought and intelligence.

The mind that controls the body is not as separated from another mind that controls another body as it appears to be.

We are all of one family. When we help ourselves, we help others. And when we help others, we help ourselves.

Good use of the body with the help of the mind contributes to the well-being of all humankind.

Do it.

Do it for your sake, and the world thanks you.

Let the neck be free, to let the head go forward and up, to let the back lengthen and widen, to let joy bring life to your body.

APPENDIX

AMERICAN CENTER
FOR THE ALEXANDER TECHNIQUE, INC.—Eastern Region
142 West End Avenue
New York, N.Y. 10023
Telephone: (212) 799-0468

AMERICAN CENTER
FOR THE ALEXANDER TECHNIQUE, INC.—
Western Region—San Francisco
931 Elizabeth Street
San Francisco, California 94114
Telephone: (415) 282-8967

AMERICAN CENTER
FOR THE ALEXANDER TECHNIQUE, INC.—
Western Region—Los Angeles
554 Rialto Avenue
Venice, California 90291
Telephone: (213) 399-3384

AMERICAN CENTER
FOR THE ALEXANDER TECHNIQUE—Mid-West Region
805 Grove Street
Glencoe, Illinois 60022
Telephone: (312) 835-0839

THE SOCIETY OF TEACHERS OF
THE ALEXANDER TECHNIQUE
3 Albert Court
Kensington Gore
London S.W.7
England

THE ALEXANDER TECHNIQUE
c/o Yehuda Kuperman
15 Rabinowitz Street
Beit Kerem
Jerusalem, Israel
(for information regarding teachers and training in Israel)

Bibliography

LISTED BELOW are the titles of books on the Alexander Technique.

Although the Technique cannot be learned from books, and only through personal instruction, these books provide background material and valuable information on the work of F. Matthias Alexander.

Barlow, Wilfred. *The Alexander Technique*. New York: Alfred A. Knopf.

Jones, Frank Pierce. *Body Awareness in Action—A Study of the Alexander Technique*. New York: Shocken, 1976.

Maisel, Edward, ed. *The Resurrection of the Body—The Essential Writings of F. Matthias Alexander*. New York: Delta Paperback.

Sherrington, C.S. *Man on His Nature*. London: Cambridge University Press, 1951.

OUT OF PRINT BOOKS (possibly available in your library)
Books by F. Matthias Alexander:
The Use Of The Self, New York: Dutton, 1932.
Man's Supreme Inheritance, New York: Dutton, 1918.
Constructive Conscious Control of the Individual, London, Methuen, 1924.
The Universal Constant in Living, New York: Dutton, 1941.

Bowden, G.C. *F. Matthias Alexander & The Creative Advance of the Individual*.

Morgan, Louise. *Inside Yourself*, London: Hutchinson, 1954.

Westfeldt, Lulie. *F. Matthias Alexander: The Man and His Work.*

References to the Alexander Technique appear in the following works:

Bonespierre: New Pathways to Piano Technique

Huxley, Aldous: End-Gaining and Means Whereby." *The Saturday Review of Literature*, October 25, 1941.

    Ends and Means.

    Eyeless in Gaza.

    Tomorrow & Tomorrow & Tomorrow

Ludovice, A.M. *Health and Education through Self-Mastery.* London: Watts & Co., 1933.

Perls, Fritz. *Ego, Hunger and Aggression*, london: Allen and Unwin, 1947 and New York: Randon House, 1969.

Shaw, George Bernard, *Shaw on Music: A Selection from the Music Criticism of Bernard Shaw.* Selected by Eric Bently. New York: Doubleday, 1955.

Sherrington, Charles S. *The Endeavor of Jean Fernal*, London: cambridge University Press, 1946.

Smith, Grover, ed. *The Letters of Aldous Huxley*, New York: Harper & Row, 1936.

Index

A

Acne, stress and, 49
Acting
    problems, solutions for, 61
    training and Alexander Technique, 62
Action, lengthening through, 195
Actors, Alexander Technique and, vii-viii, 57
Alexander, F. Matthias
    development of method by, 10
    discovery of method by, 73
    life of, ix, 73
    impact of, 79
Alexander Technique
    Centers, 126
    teacher, description of, 110
American
    Association for the Advancement of Ten-
        sion Control, 206
    Center for the Alexander Technique, 112
    Physical Fitness Research Institute, 87
Analysis of self, 15
Appearance
    change in, through Alexander Technique,
        22
Applications, institutional, of Technique,
    107
Arches, changes in, 84
Arthritis, control of, 103, 104
Asthma, control of, 103
Athletes, help for, 138
Awareness
    of body, 25, 200
    of body, increasing, 70
    increase and movement, 71
    Through Movement, Feldenkrais, 254

B

Back
    as barometer of health, 88
    exercise, special, 64
    knee exercise for, 149
    lengthening of, 18, 19
    lower, awareness of, 71
    massage, exercise for, 96
    muscles, helping, 67
    pain, alleviation of, 1, 33
    as pain source, 95
    problems and posture, 88
    problems and Technique, 87
    rigidity and sex, 46
    tension relief, 220
    upper, 220
Balance problems and Technique, 103
Barriers to success, student, 7
Bates Vision Improvement Method, 265
Baths, warm, value of, 283
Bending
    backward, avoiding, 288
    proper, 210
Benefits. See also Changes.
    of Alexander Technique, 22, 33
    in sitting, 21
Bierman, James H., writings of, 139
Bio-energetics, 252
Biofeedback, description of, 262
Blood pressure, control of, 103
Body
    awareness of, 25, 200
    awareness and joy, 130
    evaluation, 124
    habits, poor, results of, 88

language, analysis of, 249
and mind, connection of, 32
and mind integration, T'ai chi and, 59
and mind, psychological interrelationship
of, 58
and mind, relationship of. 18
misuse, pain as symptom of, 26
and personality, relationship of, 37
response to words, 179
seld-knowledge of, 163
separation, cause of, 40
signals, detecting, 117
type and personality, 18
use, poor, avoiding, 281
use, poor, tension and, 105
Books on Alexander, 76
Breathing
improvement in, 8
natural, importance of, 286
technique, 244
Bulletin of Structural Integration, 5
Bursitis, control of, 103
Business success and mental attitudes, 56

C

Calisthenics, help with, 291
Caplan, Deborah
and scoliosis, 93
writings of, 139
Carrying
a baby, 237
bags, proper way of, 234
shoulder bags, proper way of, 236
Certification of Alexander teachers, 112
Chairs
proper use of, 29
as source of body problems, 29
Changes. See also Benefits.
from Alexander Technique, 33, 34, 43, 44
in feelings, 198, 199
mental, 208
personality, 44
from stress, 243
structural, 11
Children, help for, 147
Chiropractics, description of, 258
Claims for Alexander Technique, 2
Clothing
comfortable, value of, 283
Coghill, Charles E., 79
Conditioned
reflex, 6
response, 268
Conditioning patterns, effects of, 6

Conditions that respond to Technique, 87
Consciousness
of body, increasing, 70
control, 9
Constructive thinking, 153, 154
Contraction, excess, 217
Cousins, Norman, illness experience of, 163
Coordination, improvement in, 35
Creativity and mental attitude, 56
Criminals, insane, help for, 108
Cripps, Sir Stafford, and Technique, 79

D

Daily life, application to, 5, 171
Dancers and Alexander Technique, 57
improvement for, 155, 159
Dancing
and Alexander Technique, 63, 274, 277
Defects, physical, overcoming, vii
Development of Alexander Method, 10
Dewey, John, and Technique, 79, 277
Directed movement, 123
Directing self, 116, 119, 120
Directions, Alexander. See also Words.
abbreviating the, 175
meaning of, 177
repetition of, 27
self-, 20, 175, 176, 162
Disc problems, help for, 92
Discipline of self, 110
Discovery of Alexander Technique, 73
Drama teachers and Technique, 275
Drinking habits, 229
Drug use, effects of, 242

E

Earning increase and Technique, 56
Eastern philosophies and Technique, 78
Eating habits, 229
Emotion, emotional. See also Mind,
Personality.
separation, 40
End gaining
effect of, 102
importance of, 115
Energy, intrinsic, and T'ai chi, 60
Entrance requirements for teacher training,
113
EST and Technique, 266
Exercise. See also Movement.
for back muscles, 68
back, special, 64
folding, 132
help with, 291
knee-back, 149

lying down, 166
pleasurable, 132
sitting, 188
standing, 188
Exhaustion, avoiding, 282
Eyes
and head movement, 81
keeping open, 20
use during walking, 194

F

Famous people and Alexander Technique,
79
Feelings
changes in, 198, 199
getting, 12
unusual, 198. 199
Feet, changes in, 84
Feldenkrais, Dr. Moshe
Awareness Through Movement method,
71, 137, 254
and Technique, 274
Figure improvement, 219
Force, absence in Technique of, 113, 114
Freedom through Technique, x
Functional Integration, Feldenkrais, 254

G

Gastro-intestinal problems, control of, 103
Gentleness, importance of, 69, 281
Gestalt Therapy, 253
Gravity, working with, 30, 188

H

Habits
bad, unlearning, 188
body, results of poor, 88
drinking, 229
eating, 229
postural, correction, 88
telephone holding, 229
typing, 227
writing, poor, 225
Hand
washing, proper, 224
Handwriting habits, 226
Head
correcting set of, 16
movement and eyes, 81
-neck tension, 8
proper placement of, 25
to spine, relationship of, 9
Headaches, control of, 103
Health
back as barometer of, 88
holistic, 270

mental, improving, 205
Herrigel, Eugen, writings of, 78, 161
History of Alexander Technique, ix
Home practice of Technique, 110
Huxley, Aldous, and Technique, 80
Hypnosis and Technique, 266, 267

I

Images, use of, 170
Improvement, self, 275
Inhibition, Alexander's use of word, 75
Insane criminals, help for, 108
Institute of Rehabilitation Medicine, use of
Technique at, 88
Institutional applications of Technique, 107
Integration, body
lack of, 40
Intellectuals and Technique, 80

J

Jogging, 240
Jones, Frank Pierce, book by, 76
Joy and body awareness, 130

K

Kinesthetic experience, 81
Knee-back exercise, 149
Kraus, Dr. Hans, as back specialist, 88
Kurtz, Ron, writings of, 37, 58

L

Laban Method and Technique, 274
Laughter as medicine, 163
Learning
approach of Technique, 78
language of good use, 202
Legs
stress on, 84
Leibowitz, Judith, comments of, 29, 137
Lengthening
of back, 118, 119
description of, 174, 196, 217
importance of, 138
through all action, 195
while moving, 216
Lesson
average, 125
beginning, 83
reasons for, 5
table work of, 111
Lifting heavy objects, 238
Limbs, raising, 156
Lowen, Alexander, and Bio-energetics, 252
Lower back, awareness of, 70
Lying-down exercises, 166

M

MacDonald, Patrick, comments of, 28, 30, 77

Maisel, Edward, writings of, 78, 87, 219
Martial arts, description of, 259
Massage for back, exercise for, 96
Means whereby, importance of, 115
Medical
  conditions and Technique, 101
  references for Technique, 2
Meditation, benefits of, 269
Menstrual pain, control of, 103
Mental. *See also* Mind, Thinking.
  attitude and creativity, 56
  attitude and business success, 56
  attitude, changes in, 208
  changes and sex, 48
  discipline, use of, 114
  health, improving, 205
  health problems, 105
  patients, help for, 105
Mind. *See also* Emotion, Emotional, Mental, Personality, Thinking.
  and body, psychological interrelationship of, 58
  and body, relationship of, 18, 32
  body shaping by, 37
  changes in, 197
  courses, 266
  freeing, 36
  and muscles, 56
Mirror
  self-analysis before, 15, 184-195
  working in front of, 11
Movement. *See also* Exercise.
  control of, 7
  directed and nondirected, 123
  everyday, 110, 140, 143
  of head and eyes, 81
  head, result of gentle, 81
  lessons, Technique as, 4
Moving, lengthening while, 216
Multiple sclerosis, control of, 103
Muscles
  back, helping, 67
  and mind, 56
Musicians and Technique, 57

N

Neck
  freedom, 19
  freedom, attaining, 50, 52
  tension, 8
Nerves, pinched, pain from, 96
Newman, Paul, and backaches, 61
Nondirected movement, 123
Nondoing

application of, 113
  importance of, 114, 198
Nutrition, importance of, 271

O

Observation of self, 128
Organic change, 8

P

Pain
  back, alleviation of, 1, 33
  back as source of, 95
  as body message, 94
  from pinched nerves, 96
  posture and, 74
  psychosomatic, 100
  as reason for lessons, 5
  reduction from Technique, 2, 3
  relieving others of, 296
  as symptom of body misuse, 26
Pelvic rock, 66
Perception of self, changes in, 187
Perls, Fritz, and Gestalt therapy, 253
Permanence of good use, 143
Personality. *See also* Emotion, Emotional, Mind.
  changes, 44
  stress fracture of, 41
Philosophies, Eastern, and Technique, 78
Photographs, use of, 11
Physical
  pain, effect of release from, 2
  therapy, effects on, 45
  uplift, 273
Physician, role of, 105
Physiosynthesis and Technique, 274
Physiotherapy and Technique, 273
Pleasure
  principle, importance of, 198
Poor use, avoiding, 281
Postural habits, correction of, 88
Posture
  and back problems, 88
  improvement, result of, 51
  and pain, 74
  problems, results of, vii
  and Rolfing, 257
Pregnancy and Technique, 4
Prestera, Hector, writings of, 37, 58
Primary control, 9
Problems helped by Technique, range of, 2
Psychologists and Technique, 275
Psychophysical experience, 154
Psychosomatic conditions, 100
Psychotherapy, effects on, 43, 109

R

Raising, reaching, help for, 156
Reeducation, Technique as, 6
Rehabilitation, Technique as, 71
Reichian therapy, 251
Relaxation, feeling of, 198, 270
Response, conditioned, 268
Rest breaks, 230
Resting, proper, 230
Resurrection of the Body, 78
Rolfing, 257
Running, 246
Russek, Dr. Allen, and Technique, 88

S

Saunas, value of, 283
Schools, training, 112
Scientists and Technique, 79
Scoliosis, help for, 92
Self-Alexandering, 111, 172
Self-analysis, 15
Self-directing, 116, 119, 120, 162, 175, 176
Self-experience of Technique, 64
Self-help nature of Technique, 208
Self-hypnosis and Technique, 267
Self-improvement, 275
Self-knowledge of body, 163
Self-observation, 128
Self-perception of change, 187
Self-use, 144
    proper, 5
Sensations, positive, 21
Separation, emotional, effects of, 40
Sex
    and back rigidity, 46
    life, changes in, 45
    life, improvement and Technique, 46
    and mental set, 48
Shaw, Bernard, and Technique, 79
Sherrington, Sir Charles, and Technique, 79
Shoes, comfortable, importance of, 284
Shoulder
    embrace, 220
    level, 47
Signals, body, detecting, 117
Silva Mind Control, 266
Simplicity of Technique, 24
Sitting
    benefits in, 21
    and chairs, 29
    directions for, 21
    down, 180, 182, 185
    exercise, 188
    habits, poor, 1, 23, 24
    importance of, 31

as problem cause, 28
    proper way of, 29, 144
Skin, effects of Technique on, 49
Sleep, sufficient, importance of, 285
Sleeping positions, 231
Social life, effects of Technique on, 45
Spine
    and back lengthening, 24
    head relationship to, 9
    twisting, danger of, 287
Spiritual uplift, 273
Sports, help with, 138
Standing
    exercise, 188
    habits, poor, 1
    up, 180
    up, importance of, 31
    up, proper way of, 30, 111, 184
Stress. *See also* Tension.
    and acne, 49
    appearance changes from, 243
    diseases, 87
    effects of, 36
    fracture of personality, 41
    laughter control of, 163
    reduction of physical and mental, 205-206
    release of, 50
Structural
    changes, 11
    Integration. *See* Rolfing.
Student, students
    barriers to Technique, 7
    and teacher, relationship of, 6
    variations among, 125
Stuttering, control of, 103, 104
Swimming, value of, 285

T

Table work
    exercises, 166
    at lessons, 111
T'ai chi
    and Technique, 274
    description of, 259
    and intrinsic energy, 60
Teacher, teachers
    body evaluation by, 124
    finding appropriate, 126
    role of Alexander, 10, 24, 27
    touch of, 113, 121
    trained by Alexander, 77
    training of, 112, 116
    training, entrance requirements for, 113
    variations among, 125

Telephone-holding habits, 229
Tension. *See also* Stress.
  in back, relief of, 220
  excess, 217
  head-neck, 8
  location of, 8
  and poor body use, 105
  prevalence of, 27
  reducing, 13, 14
  relief from, 4
  result of, 4, 137
  rib cage, 8
Therapy, Gestalt, 253
  physical, effects of, 45
  Reichian, 251
Thinking. *See also* Mental, Mind.
  the Alexander words, 20
  constructive, 153, 154
  control of, 14
Thomas, Milton, and Technique help, 89
Tinbergen, Professor Nikolauw, and Technique, 2, 79, 87
Torso changes, 218
Touch
  Alexander's, 78
  differences in, 122
  importance of, 11
  of teacher, 113, 121
Trainees, first Alexander, 77
Training
  of Alexander teacher, 112

excitement of, 118
mental set during, 121
process, description of, 116
schools, 112
Typing habits, 227

U

Use of the Self, The, 75

V

Vision improvement, 104
Visualization, use of, 170
Voice
  stress changes in, 243
  teachers and Technique, 275

W

Waist, reducing the, 218
Walking
  with direction, 193
  eye use during, 194
Westfeldt, Lulie, book of, 76, 116
Woodward, Joanne, and Technique, 61
Words, Alexander, 19
  thinking the, 20
  body response to, 179
Working ability and pain, relationship of, 57
Writing habits, poor, 225

Y

Yoga and Technique, 275

Z

Zen in the Art of Archery, 78, 161
Zen philosophy, Alexander and, 78